Glaucoma Update

International Glaucoma Symposium
Nara/Japan, May 7–11, 1978

Editors

G. K. Krieglstein and W. Leydhecker

With 48 Figures

Springer-Verlag Berlin Heidelberg New York 1979

Editors

Priv.-Doz. Dr. n
Professor Dr. m

Universitäts-Augen
Josef-Schneider-St

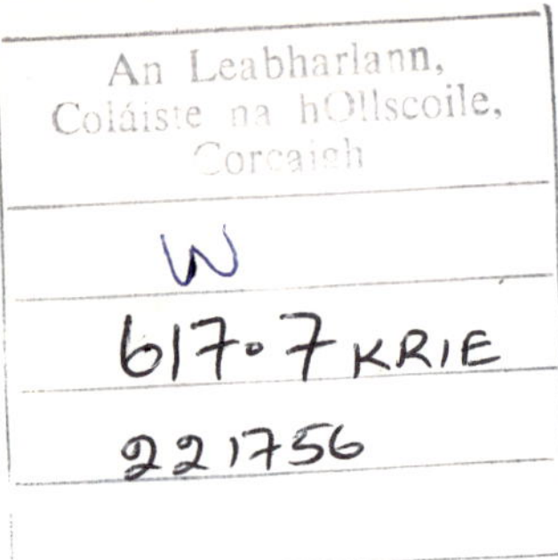

Library of Congress Cataloging in Publication Data

International Glaucoma Symposium, Nara, Japan, 1978.
Glaucoma update.

Bibliography: p. Includes index.
1. Glaucoma-Congresses. 2. Glaucoma in children-Congresses. I. Krieglstein, G. K. II. Leydhecker, Wolfgang. III. Title. [DNLM: 1. Glaucoma-Congresses. W3 IN1244 1978r / WW290 I59 1978r]
RE871.I53 1978 617.7'41 79-10747

ISBN 3-540-09350-8 Springer-Verlag Berlin Heidelberg New York
ISBN 0-387-09350-8 Springer-Verlag New York Heidelberg Berlin

Printed in Germany.

Offsetprinting and bookbinding: Konrad Triltsch, Würzburg

2127/3020–543210

International Glaucoma Symposium

Nara / Japan, May 7–11, 1978

President: W. Leydhecker

Organizers: W. Leydhecker, S. Mishima, Y. Kitazawa
in cooperation with: Japanese Glaucoma Club

Editors: G. K. Krieglstein and W. Leydhecker

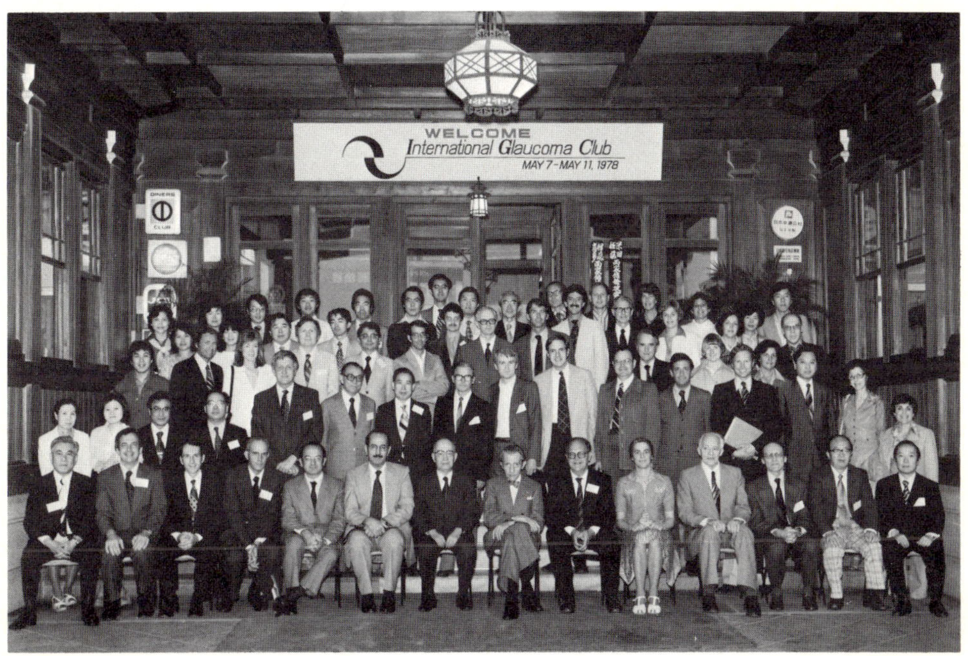

Participants of the Nara-Symposium

Acknowledgements

We are indepted to the following producers for substantial help:

Allergan Pharmaceuticals, Inc., Irvine, Ca., USA

Alza Corporation, Palo Alto, USA

American Optical Comp., West-Germany

Basotherm GmbH, Biberach, West-Germany

C.H. Boehringer Sohn, Ingelheim, West-Germany

Chibret Pharmazeutische GmbH, West-Germany

Chemie Grünenthal GmbH, Stolberg, West-Germany

Optotechnik Heine K.G., Herrsching, West-Germany

Pharm-Allergan Vetr. GmbH, Karlsruhe, West-Germany

Stierlen-Maquet AG, Rastatt, West-Germany

Dr. K. Thomae GmbH, Biberach, West-Germany

Dr. Robert Winzer, Chem.-Pharm. Fabrik, Konstanz, West-Germany

Contents

Foreword

The International Council of Ophthalmology agreed to the creation of an International Glaucoma Committee, which should have a limited number of members, 40 at a maximum. This committee will hold a closed meeting every 4 years on the occasion of the International Congress of Ophthalmology and will report to the International Council on the practical and clinical advances in glaucoma detection and treatment. This report will be published in the proceedings of the International Congress. The committee will advise and direct the activities of the International Glaucoma Society, which will hold a glaucoma symposion prior to each International Congress of Ophthalmology and which will be open to anyone interested in glaucoma.

This is now the first meeting of the committee. When I look at the program and the names of the speakers, I am convinced that it will be very fruitful. This is my most sincere wish.

I should like to thank very warmly Prof. Leydhecker for preparing the organization of this group and the scientific program and Prof. Mishima, Prof. Kitazawa, and all of their staff for having so beautifully organized this symposion, which will be very successful, and for having received us with such generous hospitality.

I am very grateful to each of the members of the International Glaucoma Committee and to each of our Japanese friends involved in this symposion.

Prof. Dr. Jules François
President of the International Council of Ophthalmology

Preface

The first meeting of the International Glaucoma Committee was held at Nara, the ancient capital of Japan. The symposium continued the tradition of similar meetings preceding the International Congress of Ophthalmology: St. Marguerithe (1954), Liège (1958), Tutzing (1966), Albi (1974). Why did all participants decide to continue such meetings in the future? There are several reasons:

We need an international forum for the discussion of a disease that still continues its sinister role in all countries, in spite of the world-wide efforts to fight it. A discussion of experts from different regions of the world will show new facets of the disease, since ophthalmological traditions, research interests, and clinical decisions differ from country to country. The discussions show to what extent differences are based on facts and to what extent on beliefs and how much they are possibly influenced by a different structure of research and of clinical medicine. Only a meeting that allots more time to discussions than it does to papers will give more opportunity for criticism than a journal or a meeting of the traditional type could do. Discussions will necessarily have an open end character, which is not pleasing to anyone who hopes for thumb rules. At our symposium, all papers were precirculated to each member, and at the meeting only a short introduction was required for each contribution, so that most of the time was free for discussions. Further advantages of this type of meeting are that: (1) very recent work can be presented and critized before publication; (2) it is possible to discuss research that gave unsatisfactory results and that one would not easily bring to the attention of a large audience; (3) prospects of research can be discussed; (4) it becomes clearer to each research worker where he will work at his best, basically or clinically; (5) the program can be kept very flexible; and (6) hopefully, efforts of different centres or individuals might be combined. By meeting each other, by talking and listening to each other, both inside and outside the lecture hall, we will succeed in understanding each other. This requires a small number of participants who live under the same roof for a few days, if possible in an area remote from the noise and distractions of a large city. This was organized at its best by Dr. Kitazawa, who did a marvelous job together with his residents and secretaries to make the meeting a full success. The thanks of all participants are also due the commercial companies who gave financial support to the meeting.

Finally, the thanks of the editors are due Springer Publishers for their co-operation in preparing this volume.

Würzburg, 12.7.78

W. Leydhecker

List of Contributors

Armaly, M.F.
George Washington University, Medical Center, Department of Ophthalmology
2150 Pennsylvania Ave., Washington, D.C. 20037, USA 131

Aulhorn, E.
University Eye Hospital
Schleichstraße 12, 7400 Tübingen, Federal Republic of Germany 79

Bengtsson, B.
University Eye Clinic, Department of exp. Ophthalmology
S-22185 Lund, Sweden 71

Calixto, N.
1177, Grão Mogol, Belo Horizonte,
Brasil 65

De Carvalho, C.A.
Rua Prof. Artur Ramos, 96 8º-and.
São Paulo-01454, Brasil 33

Draeger, J.
Augenklinik Zentralkrankenhaus
St. Jürgenstraße, 2800 Bremen, Federal Republik of Germany 205

Drance, S.M.
University of British Columbia, Department of Ophthalmology
2550 Willow Street, Vancouver, B.C. V5Z 3N9, Canada 61

Ernest, J.T.
University of Wisconsin Hospitals, Center for Health Sciences
1300 University Ave., Madison, Wisc. 53706, USA 93

Harms, H.
University Eye Hospital
Schleichstraße 12, Tübingen, Federal Republik of Germany 191

Hayreh, S.S.
University of Iowa, Department of Ophthalmology, Iowa City
Iowa 52242, USA 119

Kitazawa, Y.
University of Tokyo, School of Medicine, Department of Ophthalmology
7-3-1 Hongo, Bunkyo-Ku, Tokyo-113, Japan 169

Kolker, A.E.
Washington University, Department of Ophthalmology
660 South Euclid Ave., St. Louis, Miss. 63110, USA 11

Krasnov, M.
Director State Institute of Ophthalmology, 5 Pogodinskaja st.
Moscow-119435, USSR 201

Krieglstein, G.K.
University Eye Hospital
Josef-Schneider-Straße 11, 8700 Würzburg, Federal Republik of Germany ... 179

Kupfer, C.
National Eye Institute, National Institute of Health, Buildg. 31
9000 Rockville Pike, Bethesda, Maryland 20014, USA 27

Langham, M.E.
The Wilmer Institute, Johns Hopkins University, Ophthal. Research Unit
Baltimore, Maryland 21205, USA 19

Leopold, I.H.
University of California, California College of Medicine, Department of Ophthalmology
Irvine, Cal. 92717, USA 149

Leydhecker, W.
University Eye Hospital
Josef-Schneider-Straße 11, 8700 Würzburg, Federal Republik of Germany ... 101

Linnér, E.
University of Göteborg, Department of Ophthalmology, Sahlgren's Hospital
S-41345 Göteborg, Sweden 1

Mishima, S.
University of Tokyo, School of Medicine, Department of Ophthalmology
7-3-1 Hongo, Bunkyo-Ku, Tokyo-113, Japan 159

Podos, St.
Department of Ophthalmology, Mount Sinai Hospital
New York City, N.Y., USA 141

Sampaolesi, R.
Parana 1239.1., A-Buenos-Aires, Argentinia 39

Sears, M.L.
Yale University, School of Medicine
333 Cedar Street, New Haven, Conn. 06510, USA 153

Shaffer, R.N.
University of California, Glaucoma Clinic A 775
San Francisco, Cal. 94143, USA 53

Carboanhydrase Inhibitor Test for Early Detection of Glaucoma

Erik Linnér

University of Göteborg, Department of Ophthalmology, Sahlgren's Hospital, S-41345 Göteborg, Sweden

The term ocular hypertension is in common use when the only finding of clinical interest is an intraocular pressure that is moderately elevated above the normal range. The significance of this increase in pressure is difficult to interpret in the individual eye. FRIEDENWALD used the term normative pressure to characterize a pressure that is compatible with continued health and function for that particular eye. That pressure need not be the same in every eye. Ocular hypertension can include cases of high normative pressure but, on the other hand, also cases of early glaucoma prior to the development of detectable disk and/or field defects.

The purpose of this study is to see whether the degree of response to a carbonic anhydrase inhibitor gives useful diagnostic information. The test consists of measuring the intraocular pressure before and 3 h after a single oral dose of 500 mg (in some cases 750 mg) of acetazolamide. In the latter part of this study, conducted at the national Eye Institute, National Institutes of Health, Bethesda, Maryland, some parameters of aqueous humor dynamics were also included.

The Swedish material consisted of one group of 32 subjects with ocular hypertension. They had moderately elevated initial pressure (25.8 - 21.9 mm Hg). These subjects had been kept under clinical observation for 10 years without antiglaucomatous therapy and without evidence of progressive disk cupping or field defects. A second group consisted of 27 patients who recently had been found to have open-angle glaucoma and who had not been given any antiglaucomatous treatment. A third group consisted of 37 subjects with normotension and no history of glaucoma.

The American material consisted of 11 patients with ocular hypertension and glaucoma suspects as well as three normal volunteers. The aqueous flow before and after acetazolamide was estimated, and the residual flow was determined. The increase in ultrafiltration calculated from pseudofacility and change in pressure was included in the estimation of change in flow.

The Swedish results are summarized in Fig. 1, which shows that the percentage residual outflow pressure was 68 % in the hypertensive group as compared to approximately 50 % in the other groups. That means there is a comparatively smaller response to acetazolamide in the hypertensive group.

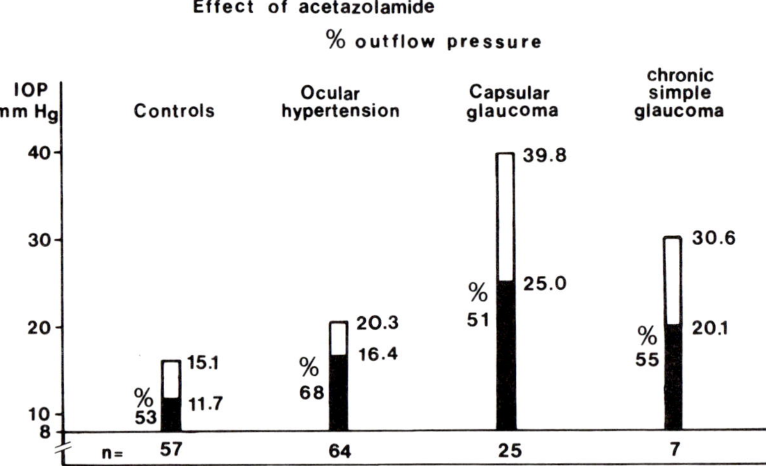

Fig.1. Normotension, hypertension, and glaucoma. The intraocular pressure and the percentage outflow pressure 3 h after an oral dose of acetazolamide. White bars before and black bars after acetazolamide.

In Fig. 2, the hypertensive and the glaucoma eyes are plotted with the initial pressure on the abscissa and the pressure 3 h after acetazolamide on the ordinate. At

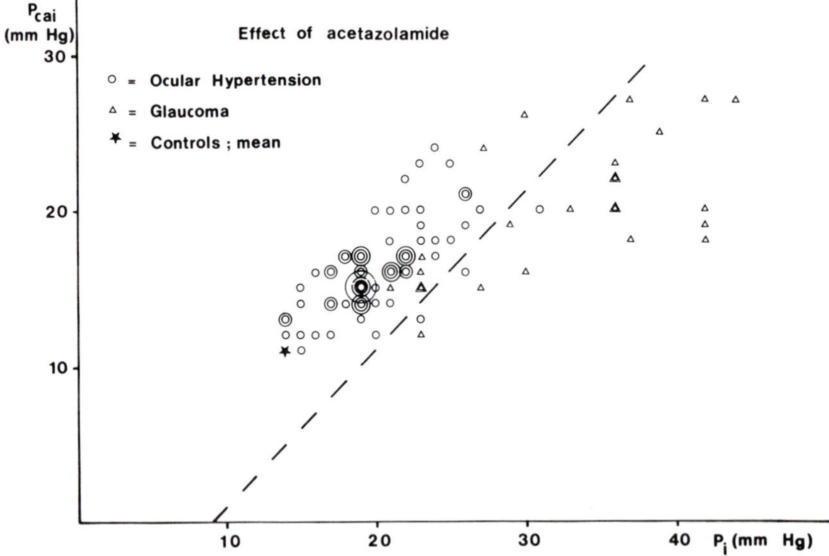

Fig.2. Ocular hypertension and glaucoma. The relationship between the intraocular pressure in the undisturbed eye (P_i) and the pressure 3 h after an oral dose of acetazolamide (P_{cai}).

moderately elevated pressure levels in the undisturbed eyes, there is a considerable overlapping between glaucomatous and hypertensive eyes. By use of this carbonic anhydrase inhibitor test, the separation between the two groups is improved although some overlapping remains.

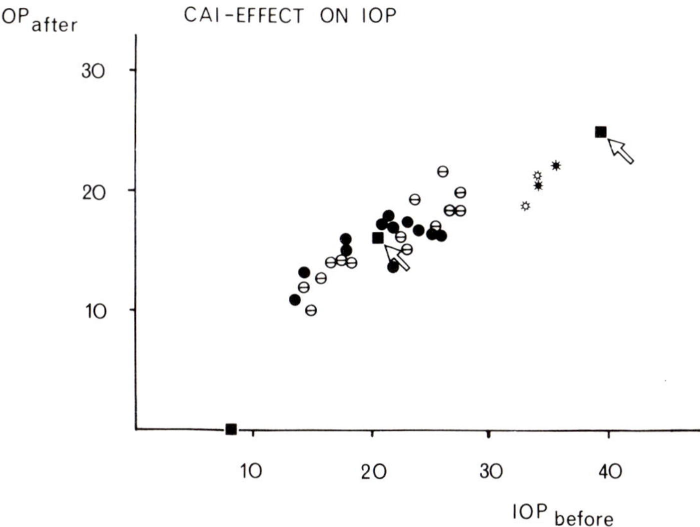

Fig.3. Preliminary American results. Normotension, ocular hypertension, and/or glaucoma suspects. The relationship between the intraocular pressure before and 3 h after an oral dose of acetazolamide. The squares indicated by arrows represent the mean values obtained in the Swedish material of ocular hypertension and glaucoma

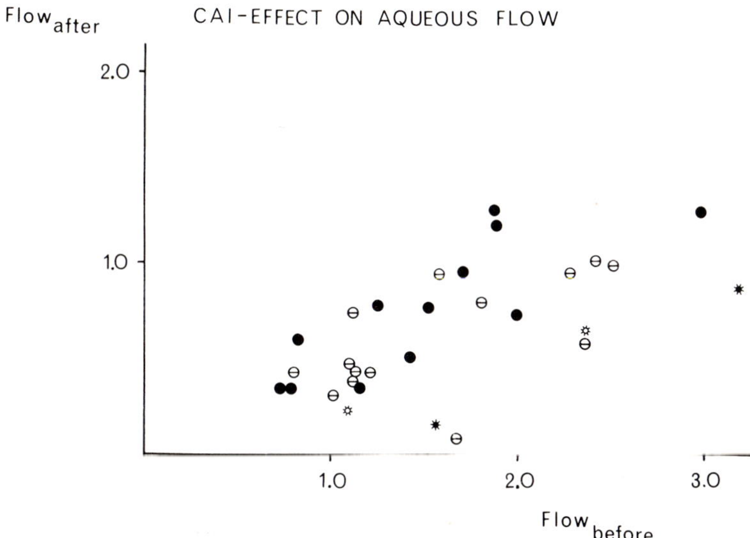

Fig.4. Preliminary American results. Normotension, ocular hypertension, and/or glaucoma suspects. The relationship between the aqueous flow before and 3 h after an oral dose of acetazolamide.

In Fig. 3, the preliminary American results are expressed as change in pressure. They are in good agreement with the results obtained in the larger Swedish group. In Fig. 4, the results from the same group of eyes in the American studies are expressed as change in aqueous flow. They indicate a similar pattern. Both in pressure response and in aqueous flow response to a carbonic anhydrase inhibitor, eyes of subjects with glaucoma appear to be more responsive than eyes of subjects with ocular hypertension.

These results must be considered as preliminary. It is necessary to perform a prospective study with a sufficient number of patients followed over a long period of time. This test can then be evaluated and its power to predict the occurrence of glaucomatous lesions determined. If the test can be limited to measuring the intraocular pressure before and after one oral dose of acetazolamide, it will be simple to perform in routine clinical work.

Reference

(1) Linnér, E.: Ocular hypertension. II. A carbonic anhydrase inhibitor test for early detection of glaucoma. Acta Ophthalmol. (in press)

Discussion

SAMPAOLESI: In your study, you have 25 eyes with pseudoexfoliation and simple glaucoma and only seven cases of simple glaucoma. Why do you use a sample so heterogeneous? In my clinical experience, simple glaucoma and pseudoexfoliation are two different diseases:

1) Pseudoexfoliation with glaucoma is usually seen in older age groups, generally 60 - 80 years of age
2) Simple glaucoma arises between 8 and 50 years of age
3) Hypertension is higher in pseudoexfoliation with glaucoma, than in chronic simple glaucoma
4) In patients with pseudoexfoliation glaucoma, there is a marked asymetry of visual field damage in both eyes
5) Frequently, there is subluxation of the lens and iridodonesis in pseudoexfoliation
6) The response to medical therapy is less marked in pseudoexfoliation than in simple glaucoma
7) The surgical complications are more frequent in pseudoexfoliation
8) Light and electron microscopy of the trabecular meshwork are quite different in the two diseases.

HALBERG: Giving 500 mg of Diamox to a person who is not under treatment with Diamox changes the osmolarity of the blood and also induces diuresis, the rate of which shows great individual differences. Unless these factors are considered, the validity of the test for clinical diagnostic purposes should be questioned. Ocular Hypertension — the term itself presents a semantic problem. I prefer: chronic glaucoma without optic nerve head disease or chronic glaucoma with optic nerve head disease. It comes down to the question: should the patient be treated or not? The term ocular hypertension tends to give false security to both the patient and the physician in an area where false security may have grave consequences for the patient.

ARMALY: I have three questions. The first refers to ocular hypertension as a concept. In the past 15 - 20 years when the practice was to treat everyone with a given pressure reading, it was useful to speak of ocular hpyertension as a state or condition in which no evidence of damage exists. Therefore, the potential harm of therapy should be weighed against the benefit. Now, long-term studies show that 45 % of those who lost fields start with a pressure of 21 or less. If we limit our concern to the hypertensives, we will be very selective and miss representing the true universe of glaucoma.

Secondly - you speak of the test results in glaucoma. Your sample includes eight eyes of open-angle glaucoma, and the majority are pseudoexfolation glaucoma. This latter differs greatly from open-angle in its vascular permeability, age, and the etiology of obstruction to outflow. Your data, therefore, should be more applicable to this group, until a larger sample of open-angle glaucoma is obtained.
The third is that the dangers of provocative tests and their usefulness has a very long tradition in ophthalmology. It is important to distinguish between the ability to separate on the basis of a test and the ability to predict the future. The latter requires a prospective study.

PHELPS: In deciding whether or not to treat a patient in an attempt to prevent visual field loss, we should consider three questions:

1) What is the probability of visual field loss?
2) What is the probability that our treatment will prevent visual field loss?
3) What are the risks and dangers of our treatment?

Our therapeutic decisions should be made in terms of probabilities, if we have sufficient data. Data regarding the probability of an individual eye developing visual field loss is only slowly accumulating. We have little information about the effectiveness of our treatment in preventing visual field loss. Finally, there is no doubt that our treatment is sometimes toxic.
It is important to remember that an eye with a high ocular pressure but a normal optic nerve does not absolutely need to have its pressure reduced, if this cannot be done easily while avoiding adverse effects of therapy. It is not necessary or desirable to use anticholinesterase miotics or surgery in these eyes. We can let the pressure remain high, rather than subject the eye to vision-threatening complications of therapy.
In the future, we should concentrate our efforts on collecting more data to help us formulate probabilities, rather than trying to identify a single test to distinguish "glaucomatous" ocular hypertension from "benign" ocular hypertension.

LEYDHECKER: Tonography is not a good method to measure aqueous secretion or aqueous flow. Do you tink that other tests for lowering the intraocular pressure, like one drop of pilocarpine 0.5%, can differentiate between ocular hypertension and beginning glaucoma? I usually give a patient with a pressure of 26 or 24 mm Hg one drop of pilocarpine 0.5%. If his pressure falls to, for example, 12 mm Hg, I think that 24 mm Hg is too much for this eye and that the normative pressure of this eye is around 12 mm Hg. If, however, the pressure comes to 21 mm Hg only after pilocarpine, I would suppose that (a) treatment is of no use and (b) the normative physiologic pressure is high and will not cause damage.

The term ocular hypertension is dangerous since it could induce young ophthalmologists to incorrectly believe that this is for all times something different from glaucoma. I would prefer the term glaucoma suspect or something similar to it, in any case a name in which the word glaucoma appears, which gives a constant warning to watch this patient further.

In practice, we have no means to predict the degree of danger in consequence of intraocular hypertension. There is no doubt that the higher the intraocular pressure, the greater the danger of visual field loss becomes, which forces us to pay the greatest attention to the intraocular pressure. It is the danger factor number one and also the danger factor that can be best measured.

There is also no doubt that there are high-risk patients who need treatment even with intraocular pressures between 20 and 25 mm Hg. There are other patients who will never need treatment with such pressures of 20 - 25 mm Hg. However, if the mean pressure of the diurnal curve exceeds 25 mm Hg, the probability of future damage to the optic nerve becomes so great that I would rather prescribe mild miotics (pilocarpine 0.5%, 3 times daily) provided that the pressure comes down below 20 and provided that this treatment is tolerated well by the patient. I think this treatment does not induce any danger to the eye.

There is no question that very strong miotics like phospholine iodide, or even an operation, should not be applied as long as the visual field is normal. I am referring only to this very mild treatment, of which I am convinced that it will not damage the eye. This seems to me better than to withhold treatment since one can never be sure that the patient will come back for many years for regular supervision. We also know that it is possible that field defects develop in a very short period of time, for example within 6 months. If untreated patients return after several years with field defects, the legal consequences would be disastrous. If such patients visited a different doctor after several years and told him that they had received no treatment in spite of increased pressures, our reputation would be in some danger.

Therefore, to summarize, I do not think there is any magic number, but usually I would rather treat patients with pressures that are constantly higher than 25 instead of waiting, unless there are special reasons that justify withholding treatment.

With pressures of 20 - 25 mm Hg, waiting is in most patients justified unless they are high-risk patients with vascular disease, a family history of glaucoma, a very large excavation, or diabetes or other risk factors. In such patients, I would rather start treatment even with pressures between 21 and 25, provided that mild miotics would lower their pressure considerably (more than 5 mm Hg).

I think that in the past there has been too much emphasis on neglecting the intraocular pressure and looking at the optic disk. The recognition of disk changes instead of paying attention to the increase of pressure is very difficult as I will show in my paper. It is also not justified just to sit back and wait until the damage occurs, because the patient with a damaged visual field is in a worse condition for treatment than the patient who still has a normal optic nerve and no field defect. The overemphasized declaration that there is no magic number has led to the neglect of pressure increases. While everyone admits that there is no magic number that would exactly differentiate between normal and pathologic cases, I think that any increase in pressure over 20 is a signal to examine and follow the patient very exactly and to think about whether and why we may withhold treatment. Withholding treatment becomes more and more risky the higher the pressure is. With pressures over 25 mm Hg, I think we are not justified in withholding mild miotics if they lower the pressure and if they are tolerated by the patients.

KOLKER: I concur with Dr. LEYDHECKER that clinically one may elect to treat those ocular hypertensives who respond to pilocarpine with a marked pressure fall. We should remember, however, that scientifically there is no evidence that demonstrates that patients so treated will do better than they would have if they had not been treated. Furthermore, there is no evidence that shows that those who respond markedly do any better or any worse than those who show little pressure response after pilocarpine administration.

SHAFFER: From the practical clinical point of view, the only aspect of chronic open-angle glaucoma over which we have control is pressure. We would all agree that the higher the pressure, the more risk there is of optic nerve damage. Therefore, I believe in a clinical trial of therapy. If pressure is markedly reduced by relatively safe medications like pilocarpine, epinephrine, or timolol and the patient is not troubled by side-effects, he should be treated.

ARMALY: I should point out that the management outlined by SHAFFER and LEYDHECKER is probably the one used by all of us.
I would like to add that the incidence of damage increases greatly with ocular pressure level. Unfortunately, ocular pressure does not predict all cases of damage. Clinically, we try to offer the patient our best judgment based on our assessment of several factors and do what we think is best. As scientists, we require the evidence to support a given recommendation.

LANGHAM: I would like to say a few words concerning the physiologic characteristics separating the ocular hypertensives and the true glaucomas. The loss of field and cupping of the disk are associated with increase of pressure and decreased outflow facility. Raised intraocular pressure does not, however, itself cause loss of visual fields, the so-called ocular hypertensives. The ocular hypertensives may themselves be divided into two subgroups; first, the systemic ocular hypertensions. This group has increased intraocular pressure due to abnormally high arterial pressure. The second group has increased intraocular pressure because their rate of aqueous humor formation is in the high range of normal. In both groups of ocular hypertensions, there is not abnormality in the pathways through which aqueous humor and blood drain.

Based on the vascular concept, the movement of a patient from the normal to the glaucoma domain may be characterized by a definite trajectory in which the position at any moment of time may be described by intraocular pressure and outflow facility. The trajectory is nonlinear. The results of LINNÉR using diamox or those of KOLKER using epinephrine are consistent with the vascular concept.

HERSCHLER: It is my belief that the only valid "predictor" we have at present to determine if damage will occur in the future is that early damage has already occurred. That is to say that more emphasis need be placed on early detection of damage to the optic nerves and/or visual field regardless of the pressure level.

A patient who presents with markedly elevated pressure but an absolutely undamaged optic nerve head has already demonstrated a resistance to damage that probably far exceeds the normal.

DRANCE: We are all in favor of finding a magic number. The problem is that we do not have any magic numbers that have stood the test of time. We know that pressure is a risk factor, and the higher it is the greater the risk. Glaucoma is, however, a complex disease and pressure is not the only factor. It makes sense that we should try to categorize the "ocular hypertensive" by many other qualities. Some belong to the dynamics of the eye but others deal with function and extraocular characteristics that will also be important. We should be looking for many magic numbers and probably an equation. Until that happens, we have clinical responsibilities and we probably manage our patients very similarly now but we should realize that much of what we do clinically does not have a factual data basis. Once parameters are recognized that possibly divide the ocular hypertensive group, they can only have meaning when they are shown prospectively as having predictive value.

Prognostic Value of Epinephrine Response

Allan E. Kolker, Michael A. Kass, Bernard Becker

Washington University, Department of Ophthalmology, 660 South Euclid Ave., St. Louis, Miss. 63110, USA

The use of topically applied epinephrine in the therapy of primary one-angle glaucoma is well-established. Recent studies suggest that the intraocular pressure response to topical epinephrine in patients with ocular hypertension may also have predictive value in determining which of such patients will develop glaucoma. The present paper reviews some of these studies, emphasizes certain of their limitations, and outlines plans to verify the conclusions suggested by the data.

BECKER and MORTON (2) demonstrated that unilateral topical epinephrine therapy in patients with ocular hypertension could prevent the development of visual field loss in the treated eyes. Subsequently, a long-term study was undertaken to determine if lowering of intraocular pressure in one eye of ocular hypertensive subjects would provide protection against the development of glaucomatous damage. Nineteen patients with symmetric ocular hypertension, normal visual fields, and symmetric optic cups were treated for 1 - 5 years (mean 3 + years) with 1 % or 2 % epinephrine HCl twice daily to one eye. (15) The characteristics of the 19 patients are summarized in Table 1. The mean age of the patients was 56 years; 32 % had a family history of glaucoma, 11 % were known diabetics, and the length of follow-up prior to epinephrine therapy was 4 years with a range of 1 - 12 years. The mean pressure differential between the epinephrine-treated eyes and the fellow eyes was 6.3 mm Hg. The project was designed so that patients who did not develop a fall in intraocular pressure while receiving epinephrine therapy were dropped from the study. The mean baseline intraocular pressure was 27 mm Hg, and the mean baseline cup/disk ratio was 0.45.

Visual field defects developed in 32 % of the untreated eyes and in none of the treated eyes. Progressive cupping, documented by disk photographs, occurred in 53 % of the fellow eyes and in 11 % of the epinephrine-treated eyes. Either visual field defects and/or progressive cupping was found in 58 % of the fellow eyes, as opposed to 11 % of the treated eyes (Table 2). Claucomatous damage was more frequent in subjects followed for more than 3 years and in the patients with a cup/disk ratio $\geqslant 0.4$. None of the eyes, either treated or untreated, with mean intraocular pressures less than 24 mm Hg developed damage in this series. Progressive cupping was observed prior to or in association with visual field defects in most cases.

Table 1.—Information on 19 Selected Patients With Ocular Hypertension

Mean age, yr	56.4 ± 12.8
Family history of glaucoma	6 of 19 subjects (32%)
Diabetes mellitus	2 of 19 subjects (11%)
Length of follow-up for ocular hypertension before unilateral epinephrine study	1 to 12 yr (mean 4 yr)
Male to female ratio	12:7
White to black ratio	13:6
Mean baseline IOP, OD, mm Hg	27.0 ± 3.5
Mean baseline IOP, OS, mm Hg	27.3 ± 3.2
Mean baseline horizontal cup/disc ratio, OD	0.45 ± 0.19
Mean baseline horizontal cup/disc ratio, OS	0.44 ± 0.18
Mean baseline IOP ⩾ 30 mm Hg	10 of 38 eyes (26%)
Spontaneous peak baseline IOP ⩾ 30 mm Hg	28 of 38 eyes (74%)

Table 2.—Development of Glaucomatous Damage

	No. Eyes	Development of Visual Field Defect	Progressive Cupping	Development of Visual Field Defect and/or Progressive Cupping
Untreated eyes	19	6 (32%)	10 (53%)	11 (58%)
Epinephrine-treated eyes	19	0 (0%)	2 (11%)	2 (11%)
		$P < .05$	$P < .025$	$P < .01$

Source: SHIN et al. (15)

The high incidence of visual field loss (32%) among the patients in this study was unexpected and rather disturbing. Numerous studies of patients with ocular hypertension demonstrate that the likelihood of visual field loss without treatment is less than 10% in periods of 5 - 10 years. (1,7-9, 12, 14, 18) It was felt that the relatively older age of the subjects, the higher intraocular pressure, the longer duration of ocular hypertension, the large cup/disk ratio, and the high incidence of a family history of glaucoma might all play a role in the results. The possibility that unilateral epinephrine might alter the perfusion of the optic nerve in the fellow eye without a decrease in intraocular pressure and thereby tend to make it more vulnerable to visual field loss was also considered. Nevertheless, none of these factors appeared to fully explain the high incidence of visual field loss in the untreated fellow eyes. SHIN (15) suggested that the patients dropped from the unilateral study because they failed to develop a fall in intraocular pressure be further evaluated. He found that these less responsive patients to topical epinephrine had a far better prognosis in regard to the development of visual field loss. None of the patients dropped from the study because of a failure to respond to topical epinephrine developed glaucomatous visual field loss during the period of the study. This suggested that the intraocular pressure response to topical epinephrine might have predictive value for the development of glaucoma among patients with ocular hypertension.

The records of 80 ocular hypertensive patients who were high responders (GG) to topical corticosteroids (intraocular pressure ⩾ 31 mm HG after 6 weeks of topical dexamethasone 0.1 % q.i.d.) were evaluated. (3) These subjects had been treated for various reasons with topical epinephrine twice daily to one eye for periods of 24 or seven days. All subjects had been followed for 5 - 10 years and at least one eye was untreated during the entire period. A response to topical epinephrine was defined as a decrease of > 5 mm Hg in the treated eye, corrected for any change in the untreated eye. Twenty of the 80 ocular hypertensive subjects developed visual field loss during the follow-up period. Seventeen of the 20 (85 %) were responders to topical epinephrine, as opposed to 17 of 60 (28 %) of the subjects who maintained normal visual fields. Furthermore, the incidence of visual field loss was 50 % (17/34 eyes) in epinephrine responders as opposed to 6.5 % (3/46 eyes) in the non-responders. Intraocular pressure response to topical epinephrine was a better prognostic indicator of the development of glaucoma than the initial intraocular pressure. This suggested the practical and clinically very important possibility that epinephrine could be used as a prognostic test in patients with ocular hypertension and enable the clinician to predict which patients were most vulnerable to the development of visual field loss.

Before accepting the above conclusions, several aspects of thedata presented must be carefully considered. The studies were retrospective and require prospective confirmation; they were done in one center and in only one population group; the patients were highly selected and the conclusions may or may not apply to other patients. The subjects had rather marked ocular hypertension, were high responders to topical corticosteroids, had a high frequency of a family history of glaucoma, had large cup/disk ratios and poor outflow facilities by tonography. For all of these reasons, the findings must be confirmed in less select populations before the conclusions can be accepted. Prospective studies of epinephrine responsiveness in patients with ocular hypertension are in progress but will require a number of years before the results are available.

Other aspects of epinephrine responsiveness have been investigated. For example, the intraocular pressure response to topically applied epinephrine was found to be similar at 4 h, 24 h, and 7 days. (6) In a mixed group of ocular normotensive and ocular hypertensive subjects, the mean intraocular pressure response at 4 h and at 24 h was similar, with a correlation coefficient of 0.6. This suggested that future tests of epinephrine responsiveness could be done more conveniently in a 4 h period with the medication instilled by the observer rather than depending upon the patient to use medication.

The mean corrected intraocular pressure response in 35 ocular normotensive subjects was 2.9 mm Hg (18.8% of the baseline IOP), in 62 ocular hypertensive subjects 3.7 mm Hg (16.8% of the baseline IOP), and in 27 primary open-angle glaucoma subjects 7.3 mm Hg (25.4% of the baseline IOP) (KAAS, unpublished). This suggests that the response is similar in ocular normotensive and ocular hypertensive subjects with the greater response in ocular hypertensives a reflection of the higher starting intraocular pressure. In patients with primary open-angle glaucoma, however, there was both a greater absolute and a greater relative intraocular pressure response.

Epinephrine responsiveness was tested and compared in 16 patients with primary open-angle glaucoma and 16 patients with secondary glaucoma, (4) matched for age, sex, race, prevalence of vascular disease, and duration of therapy and initial intraocular pressure. 14 of 16 patients (88%) with primary open-angle glaucoma had corrected intraocular pressure responses to topical epinephrine of > 5 mm Hg, compared to 5 of 16 (31%) of the patients with secondary glaucoma. In addition, while on treatment with topical epinephrine, 11 of the subjects with primary open-angle glaucoma had one or more premature ventricular contractions per 4 min tonogram as opposed to three of the secondary glaucoma patients. This suggests that patients with primary open-angle glaucoma are more sensitive to the effects of epinephrine systemically as well as in the eye.

PALMBERG (13) has recently demonstrated that lymphocytes from patients with primary open-angle glaucoma are more sensitive to epinephrine-induced inhibition of lymphocyte transformation than are the lymphocytes from normal individuals. Corticosteroids have been shown to inhibit lymphocyte transformation, (5, 11) and c-AMP appears to have much the same effect. (16) Since epinephrine is known to raise the level of c-AMP in many tissues including the eye, (10, 17) one can postulate that patients with primary open-angle glaucoma tend to have a greater accumulation of, or perhaps and increased reaction to, c-AMP compared with nonglaucomatous patients. The systemic and ocular hyperresponsiveness to epinephrine could be explained by such a hypothesis.

Summary.

The possible prognostic implications for the development of primary open-angle glaucoma among ocular hypertensive patients responsive to topical epinephrine are reviewed. Subjects whose intraocular pressures fall more than 5 mm Hg appear to be particularly prone to later development of glaucoma. Epinephrine testing may be of considerable importance in the clinical management and follow-up of patients with ocular hypertension. The need for confirmation of these preliminary and retrospective studies is emphasized.

Reverences

(1) Armaly, M.F.: Ocular pressure and visual fields: A ten year follow-up study. Arch. Ophthalmol. 81, 25 (1969)

(2) Becker, B.; Morton, W.R.: Topical epinephrine in glaucoma suspects. Am. J. Ophthalmol. 62, 272 (1966)

(3) Becker, B.; Shin, D.H.: Response to topical epinephrine: A practical prognostic test in patients with ocular hypertension. Arch. Ophthalmol. 94, 2057 (1976)

(4) Becker, B.; Montgomery, S.W.; Kass, M.A.: Increased ocular and systemic responsiveness to epinephrine in primary open-angle glaucoma. Arch. Ophthalmol. 95, 789 (1977)

(5) Bigger, J.F.; Palmberg, P.F.; Becker, B.: Increased cellular sensitivity to glucocorticoids in primary open-angle glaucoma. Invest. Ophthalmol. 11, 832 (1972)

(6) Kass, M.A.; Becker, B.: A simplified test of epinephrine responsiveness. Arch. Ophthalmol. (in press) (1978)

(7) Kitazawa, Y.: Problems on primary open-angle glaucoma. Acta Soc. Ophthalmol. Jpn. 79, 1715 (1975)

(8) Linner, E.: Diagnostic and therapeutic aspects of early chronic simple glaucoma. Isr. J. Med. Sci. 8, 1394 (1972)

(9) Linner, E.; Stromberg, U.: Ocular hypertension. In: Glaucoma Symposium, Tutzing Castle. Leydhecker, W. (ed.), p. 187. Basel: Karger 1967

(10) Neufeld, A.H.; Jampol, L.M.; Sears, M.L.: Cyclic AMP in the aqueous humor: The effects of adrenergic action. Exp. Eye Res. 14, 242 (1973)

(11) Newell, P.C.: Inhibition of human leukocyte mitosis by prednisolone in vitro. Cancer Res. 21, 1518 (1961)

(12) Norskov, K.: Routine tonometry in ophthalmic practice: II. Five year follow-up. Acta Ophthalmol. 48, 873 (1970)

(13) Palmberg, P.F.; Hajeck, S.; Cooper, D.; Becker, B.: Increased cellular responsiveness to epinephrine in primary open-angle glaucoma. Arch. Ophthalmol. 95, 855 (1977)

(14) Perkins, E.S.: The Bedford Glaucoma Survey: 1. Long-term follow-up of borderline cases. Br. J. Ophthalmol. 57, 179 (1973)

(15) Shin, D.H.; Kolker, A.E.; Kass, M.A.; Kaback, M.B.; Becker, B.: Long-term epinephrine therapy of ocular hypertension. Arch. Ophthalmol. 94, 2059 (1976)

(16) Smith, J.W.; Steiner, A.L.; Newberry, W.M., et al: Cyclic adenosine 3'5'-monophosphate in human lymphocytes. Alteration after phytohemagglutinin stimulation. J. Clin. Invest. 50, 432 (1971)

(17) Sutherland, E.W.; Øye, I.; Butcher, R.W.: The action of epinephrine and the role of adenylcyclase system in hormone action. Recent Prog Horm. Res. 21, 623 (1965)

(18) Wilensky, J.T.; Podos, S.M.; Becker, B.: Prognostic indicators in ocular hypertension. Arch. Ophthalmol. 91, 200 (1974)

Discussion

PHELPS: In a recent study performed jointly at the glaucoma clinics of Duke University and the University of Iowa, 38 patients were treated with epinephrine for 3 weeks. Eleven patients had glaucomatous visual field loss in at least one eye. Twenty-seven patients had no visual field loss.

The percentage reduction of ocular pressure was 20.4 % in the glaucoma group and 20.9 % in the group with ocular hypertension. The frequency with which ocular pressure fell by 6 mm Hg or greater was 60 % in those with visual field loss and 50 % in those without. This difference was not statistically significant. These results suggest that patients susceptible to glaucomatous damage are not preferentially hypersensitive to epinephrine.

DRANCE: We were hoping to reproduce the epinephrine study, for it would have simplified the management of ocular hypertension. We therefore tested untreated open-angle glaucoma patients and untreated ocular hypertensives. We performed the epinephrine tests exactly in the way described by the St. Louis group. Unfortunately, in the glaucoma group, 10 of 18 (56 %) showed a positive epinephrine response and in the ocular hypertensive group 17 of 32 (53 %) showed a positive response. These differences are not statistically significant. If this test were predictive, one would have expected the glaucoma group to have a much higher prevalence of positive responses. If this test is to have any clinical significance, a prospective study will have to establish this difference, but at the moment our findings suggest that it does not have such predictive value and in fact the epinephrine pressure reduction is related to the height of the initial pressure.

ZIMMERMAN: Drs. DRANCE and PHELPS found the same incidence of the "epi-response" ocular hypertension as in glaucoma.

I must admit that the data from Drs. DRANCE and PHELPS blunts my enthusiasm that the epi-responsiveness test will turn out to be a predictive means of separating those ocular hypertensive patients who will go on to glaucoma from those who will not. Their hypothesis that there should be a much higher percentage of epi-responders in the glaucoma group as compared to the ocular hypertension group is sound. On the other hand, Dr. KOLKER has demonstrated that the epi-response test can separate the ocular hypertensive patients into two groups, and his preliminary evidence suggests that these groups may in fact be different pertaining to field loss. Ocular hypertensive patients are different from glaucoma patients, and it is conceivable that many things (parameters) change when a patient slowly progresses from ocular hypertension to glaucoma. Regardless of the retrospective data or hypothesis at this point, the "proof of the pudding" is a prospective study. Dr. KOLKER has shown us a method for further separating and characterizing the ocular hypertensive patient, which should be recorded for every ocular hypertensive patient and then the predictability of this test will become apparent.

LEYDHECKER: How would you explain the difference between your results and those of DRANCE and PHELPS?

MISHIMA: (1) Is there any difference in the glaucoma family history between the epinephrine responders and nonresponders? (2) I wonder if the diversity of the results among three reporters (KOLKER, DRANCE, and PHELPS) had to do with the borderline you draw, i.e., 5 mm Hg. Was there a skew in the distribution of the epinephrine response that leads to setting the line at this Level?

KRIEGLSTEIN: Different responses might occur if you did not use the same epinephrine preparation throughout your study, since come preparations contain benzalkonium chloride and others do not. In this respect, you might have a different rate of penetration of the drug in the different groups of patients.

HERSCHLER: Had these primary open-angle glaucoma patients been under treatment prior to epinephrine testing? If so, how long had therapy been stopped prior to epinephrine testing?

ERNEST: Is it possible that epinephrine applied to one eye might be systemically absorbed and cause a deterioration in visual field in the fellow eye and thus account for the results of your study?

PODOS: As the epinephrine responders have a higher mean baseline pressure than the nonresponders, even though you analyzed the data in two pressure groups, high and low, and still found differences, it becomes clear that at least some of the differences are due to initial intraocular pressure level. Eyes with higher pressure achieve a greater reduction from any drug in terms of absolute mm Hg.

Adrenoceptor Mechanisms in the Outflow Channels of Normal and Glaucomatous Eyes

Maurice E. Langham

The Johns Hopkins University, Ophthal. Research Unit, Baltimore, Maryland 21205, USA

Norepinephrine is synthesized and stored in the terminals of the adrenergic neuronal network that innervate the iris, the ciliary processes, and the channels draining the aqueous humor (3). The release of norepinephrine from presynaptic sites results in an interaction with specific membrane receptors, and it is the molecular configuration of these adrenergic receptors that determines their structural specificity. This molecular specificity also determines the pharmacologic activity of both adrenoceptor agonists and antagonists. This paper deals with our present knowledge of the adrenergic receptor mechanism that modulate the flow resistance of the outflow channels in normal and glaucomatous eyes.

Postsynaptic α- and β-adrenoceptors. Stimulation of α-adrenoceptors by the topical application of adrenoceptor agonists results in rapid pupil dilatation and a slow onset of decreased intraocular pressure (IOP) and outflow resistance in rabbits and man. These responses are specific to the α-adrenergic receptor and may be blocked by the appropriate α-adrenoceptor blocking agents (10, 14).

With repeated stimulation of the α-adrenoceptors, biphasic responses of both IOP and outflow resistance develop. This has been observed in normal and glaucomatous eyes and in rabbits using norepinephrine and the mixed agonist, epinephrine. Both the ocular hypotensive and the hypertensive responses and the associated changes in outflow resistance are mediated by the α-adrenoceptors and are blocked by the specific α-antagonists (5, 12).

The importance of the adrenergic neural innervation to these α-adrenoceptor responses is dramatically illustrated in 2-3 log increase in response sensitivity to α-adrenoceptor agonists after surgical excision of the superior cervical ganglion (2, 7).

The presence of β_2-adrenoceptors in the outflow channels is well-established, based on the analysis of the ocular response to β-adrenoceptor agonists and antagonists. The highly selective β_2-agonist, salbutamol, has intense vasodilator properties, and when applied topically, it causes a rapid decrease of IOP and outflow resistance. These responses are blocked by prior administration of β-adrenoceptor antagonists (11). A more specific type of β-blockade is shown by the ability of timolol but not atenolol to block the ocular responses to salbutamol. Timolol acts primarily on β_2-sites, whereas atenolol acts primarily on β_1-sites. There is no evidence that β_1-sites are present in the outflow mechanism.

The specific vasodilator β_2-adrenoceptor agonists and those catecholamines having mixed but dominantly β-agonist activity will induce biphasic changes in IOP and outflow resistance when applied repeatedly to the eye (11). As with the α-adrenoceptor agonists, both aspects of the biphasic response are blocked by timolol and less specific β-blocking agents, including propranolol.

In the chronic administration of β_2-adrenoceptor agonists including the mixed α, β-agonists, the increase of IOP and outflow resistance induced by the β-agonist may overshadow completely the favorable hypotensive response. Thus, in the therapeutic use of mixed agonists including epinephrine, the addition of the β_2-blocking agent, timilol, increases the pressure and outflow resistance responses to epinephrine (LANGHAM, unpublished observations).

<u>The structural interdependence of the α- and β-adrenoceptor sites.</u> The two receptor sites operate independently to a major degree. Blockade of the α-receptors by the appropriate antagonists leaves free the ability of the remaining β-sites to respond to the β_2-agonist (LANGHAM, unpublished observation). Similarly, the biphasic pressure response to an α-agonist does not modify the qualitative nature of the response to the β-agonists.

<u>Presynaptic α_2-adrenoceptor sites and central neural adrenergic actions on IOP.</u> Recent pharmacologic studies of the comparative actions of the α-adrenoceptor agonists norepinephrine and clonidine on IOP have indicated the presence of two types of α-adrenoceptors. Norepinephrine stimulates the α_1-subclasses, which are postsynaptic, whereas clonidine acts weakly at these sites. However, clonidine has a greater affinity for the α_2-sites that act presynaptically and mediate a negative feedback control of norepinephrine release.

Clonidine applied topically causes a rapid decrease of IOP but has little mydriadic effect. Unlike norepinephrine, which causes increase in the outflow facility, clonidine has little effect on the outflow facility. Its ocular hypotensive action is due predominantly to decrease of the rate of aqueous humor formation.

Clonidine is an extremely interesting and important drug in that it provides one of the first examples of an ocular hypotensive drug whose action is dependent on both peripheral and central neural actions (1, 6). The central nervous response is due to stimulation of α-adrenoceptors of the vasomotor centers of the medulla oblongata, which causes a general decrease of efferent sympathetic nerve activity to the peripheral organs. The central neural ocular hypotensive action mediated by the adrenergic nerves has been confirmed by the observation that the central effect of clonidine on intraocular pressure is dependent on an intact adrenergic innervation of the eye (1). In this respect, it is of fundamental significance that the β_2-blocker timolol also has peripheral and central neural actions on IOP and that its central effect is mediated by the adrenergic innervation of the eye (9). In this respect, it is pertinent that both clonidine and timolol have similar actions on aqueous humor dynamics; both have little, if any effect on the outflow resistance, but both decrease the rate of aqueous humor formation.

Adenyl cyclase and the cyclic nucleotides. The cyclic nucleotides, adenosine cyclic 3'5' monophosphate (AMP) and guanosine cyclic 3,5']' monophosphate (GMP) have been shown to regulate innumerable biologic processes. Of pertinence to the present problem is the establishment that cyclic nucleotides mediate the actions of adrenergic agonists and influence smooth muscle vasomotor tone.

Adenyl cyclase, the enzyme that catalyzes the conversion of ATP to AMP, consists of a catalytic subunit facing the interior of the cell. Adrenergic agonists and antagonists are thought to interact with specific receptor sites present only in the cell membranes. It is the variation in the properties of the receptor rather than that of the activity of the adenyl cyclase that is responsible for the specificity of the response.

In the eye, it is evident that both α- and β-adrenergic agonists increase c-AMP and stimulate adenyl cyclase. This occurs not only in those tissues innervated by adrenergic neurones but also in the noninnervated structures including the crystalline lens. The action of adrenergic α- and β-agonists on IOP is associated with increase of c-AMP in the aqueous humor, and it has been suggested that c-AMP itself might mediate decreased outflow resistance (15). In support of this view, it has been shown that abnormally high concentrations of c-AMP and several analogues such as dibutyl-cAMP and 8 methothio 3'5'-AMP cause decrease of the outflow resistance when injected into the rabbit anterior chamber (16).

Subsequent studies, however, show that the extracellular c-AMP is unlikely to directly influence outflow facility. Thus, c-AMP concentrations in the aqueous humor have failed to correlate with IOP change (17). For example, the increase of c-AMP in the aqueous humor following topical administration of norepinephrine, epinephrine, and isoproterenol is associated with both phases of the biphasic responses in pressure and outflow facility.

It may be concluded that the ocular response to adrenergic agonists is mediated by the adenyl cyclase system, but that extracellular cAMP plays little if any role in the response of the outflow system to adrenergic compounds.

The physiologic implications of these findings. Interpretation of the response of the outflow system to adrenergic drugs is based on recent clarification of the principal morphologic and hydrodynamic features of the drainage channels. These channels form a series of two communicating networks, an inner trabecular meshwork of small channels and an outer intrascleral plexus of larger channels that are well-separated in man and primates by the canal of Schlemm (4, 8, 13, 14).

The channels of the intrascleral venous plexus may be divided into three categories depending on whether they are filled with blood, with aqueous humor, or with a mixture of blood and aqueous humor. Experimental and mathematic analyses of flow through the outflow system in dead and living eyes have established that the outflow resistance of the living eye is significantly greater than that of the dead eye and several times greater than that of the trabecular meshwork.

The ability of α- and β-adrenoceptor agonists to cause biphasic changes of the IOP and of the outflow resistance finds explanation in the integration of the responses of each component part of the outflow channels. As a working hypothesis, it was proposed that increase of IOP and outflow resistance induced by α-adrenoceptor agonists results from vasoconstriction of the aqueous and episcleral veins and that decrease of IOP and outflow resistance are due to vasoconstriction of the blood supply to the intrascleral plexus. Much experimental and clinical research in animals and in normal and glaucomatous human eyes is consistent with this concept (8, 13).

References

(1) Allen, R.C.; Langham, M.E.: The intraocular pressure response of conscious rabbits to clonidine. Invest. Ophthalmol. 15, 815-823 (1976)

(2) Eakins, K.E.; Tyan, S.J.: The action of sympathomimetic amines on the outflow of aqueous humor from the eye. J. Pharmacol. 23, 374-382 (1964)

(3) Ehinger, B.: Adrenergic nerves to the eye and to related structures in man and in Cynomolgus monkey (Macaca irus). Invest. Ophthalmol. 5, 45-52 (1966)

(4) Hart, R.W.: Theory of neural mediation of intraocular dynamics. Bull. Math. Biol. 34, 113-40 (1972)

(5) Krieglstein, G.K.; Langham, M.E.: The biphasic intraocular pressure and outflow facility responses of normal and glaucomatous eyes to epinephrine. Albrecht von Graefes Arch. Klin. Ophthalmol. (in press) (1978)

(6) Krieglstein, A.K.; Langham, M.E.; Leydhecker, W.: The peripheral and central actions of clonidine in normal and glaucomatous eyes. Invest. Ophthalmol. 17, 149-158 (1978)

(7) Langham, M.E.: The response of the pupil and intraocular pressure of conscious rabbits to adrenergic drugs following unilateral superior cervical ganglionectamy. Exp. Eye Res. 4, 381-389 (1965)

(8) Langham, M.E.: The aqueous outflow system and its response to autonomic receptor agonists. Exp. Eye Res. 25, 311-322 (1977)

(9) Langham, M.E.; Craigie, B.: The paradoxical effects of adrenoceptor agonists and antagonists on intraocular pressure. Proceedings of the A.R.V.O. Meeting. Sarosota, 1978

(10) Langham, M.E.; Diggs, E.M.: Qantitative studies of the ocular responses to norepinephrine. Exp. Eye Res. 13, 161-171 (1972)

(11) Langham, M.E.; Diggs, E.M.: Adrenergic responses in the eyes of rabbits, primates and man. Exp. Eye Res. 19, 281-95 (1974)

(12) Langham, M.E.; Krieglstein, G.K.: The biphasic intraocular pressure response of rabbits to epinephrine. Invest. Ophthal. 15, 119-127 (1976)

(13) Langham, M.E.; Palewicz, K.: The pupillary, the intraocular pressure, and the vasomotor responses to norepinephrine. J. Physiol. (Lond.) 267, 339-55 (1977)

(14) Langham, M.E.; Diggs, E.M.: Adrenergic responses in the eyes of rabbits, primates and man. Exp. Eye Res. 19, 281-95 (1974)

(15) Neufeld, A.H.; Jampol, L.M.; Sears, M.L.: Cyclic AMP in the aqueous humor: The effects of adrenergic agents. Exp. Eye Res. 14, 242-50 (1972)

(16) Neufeld, A.H.; Dueker, D.K.; Sears, M.L.: Cyclic AMP and outflow facility. Paper presented at the A.R.V.O. Meeting. Sarasota, 1974

(17) Radius, R.; Langham, M.E.: Cyclic AMP and the ocular responses to norepinephrine. Exp. Eye Res. 17, 219-29 (1973)

Discussion

LEYDHECKER: Do all vessels, of which you said that they contract or dilate, have muscles?

KRIEGLSTEIN: You stated that there are no β_1-receptors in the eye. We tried metoprolol, which is supposed to be one of the most selective β_1-blockers, and we got a beautiful IOP decrease. How can you explain that?

LANGHAM: The evidence for β_1-adrenoceptors is restricted to cardiac muscle. The ability of atenolol and bupranolol to decrease intraocular pressure may reflect their nonspecific action including an ability to block β_2-receptors at higher concentrations than they block β_1-receptors.

BILL: As to the site of the outflow resistance, I feel that the biphasic pressure response to α-adrenoceptor agonists could be explained on the view that the trabecular meshwork was the site of major flow resistance. I feel that the prolonged ocular hypotensive response could be attributed to a direct effect on the trabecular meshwork and that the transient hypertensive response could be attributed to vasoconstriction of the episcleral vessels and increased episcleral pressure.

LANGHAM: I would like to point out that the biphasic pressure response to α-adrenoceptor agonists and to β_2-adrenoceptor agonists were associated with biphasic changes in outflow resistance, a parameter independent of episcleral venous pressure. Furthermore, the location of major outflow resistance in the intrascleral venous plexus where blood and aqueous humor compete for the same channels has been established by direct experimental procedures.

ZIMMERMAN: I think that the rabbit is a useless animal for studying adrenergic pharmacology of the eye and that all results were of no value.

LANGHAM: I disagree strongly with this view. Qualitatively, the adrenoceptor responses in the eyes of rabbits and man have been found to be the same in all instances, which had been stressed in may own studies in which both rabbits and man had been compared.

HAYREH: I am not clear about Dr. LANGHAM 'S explanation. As fars as I can understand, he implies that vascular disturbances in the anterior segment and those in the optic nerve head are related to one another. I find it hard to follow the logic since the two vascular systems are totally different, and, moreover, the disturbances in the anterior segment are presumably in the aqueous veins while those in the posterior segment are in arterial supply. Since he postulates that both types of vascular disturbances may be secondary to collagen disorders in the sclera, i.e., in the trabecular meshwork anteriorly and the lamina cribosa posteriorly, glaucoma thus becomes essentially a collagen disorder instead of being a vascular disorder — we have little evidence to support this hypothesis. I have all along, in the past, strongly stressed that results of ophthalmic research from the rabbit should not be carried over to the human because of gross anatomic differences between man and rabbit, let alone the physiologic differences. For example, rabbits have a very different type of anterior segment, with no canal of Schlemm and poorly developed ciliary muscle. In the posterior segment, rabbits do not have lamina cribrosa, the anatomy of the optic nerve is different, and the retina is mostly avascular in them. Thus, I would make a strong plea that ophthalmic research should not be carried out in the rabbit as far as possible since the results cannot be carried over from the rabbit to man.

New Hypothesis on Anterior Chamber Developmental Anomalies Associated with Glaucoma

Carl Kupfer

National Eye Institute, National Institute of Health, Buildg. 31,
9000 Rockville Pike, Bethesda, Maryland 20014, USA

A most interesting group of congenital and developmental anomalies is that involving the structures forming the anterior chamber. In these anomalies, the cornea, iris, or trabecular meshwork are affected to varying degrees, and often there are elevations of intraocular pressure. A number of eponyms have been used for these malformations such as Axenfeld's anomaly, Rieger's anomaly, and Peter's anomaly, as well as descriptive terms such as goniodysgenesis associated with hereditary juvenile glaucoma. Collectively, this group of conditions have been referred to as the anterior chamber cleavage syndrome. (10)

At present, the pathogenesis of this group of diseases is thought to be a developmental defect in the migration of the paraxial mesoderm, which was believed to form the corneal stroma and endothelium as well as the superficial iris stroma, while persistence of mesodermal tissue in the angle due to faulty or incomplete cleavage of the anterior chamber was thought to contribute to the increased outflow resistance and glaucoma. (1, 2)

There are several problems relating to this hypothesis. It is difficult to explain the extensive spectrum of clinical findings in which almost every combination and permutation of involvement of the cornea (sclerocornea, megalocornea, corneal opacities, endothelial dystrophy), or iris and pupil (hypoplasia of the iris stroma, iris adhesions to cornea, corectopia, pseudopolycoria, dyscoria), or anterior chamber angle (fine iris strands or iris adhesions to the trabecular meshwork and/or cornea) occur to some degree. Secondly, there does not appear to be a good correlation between the presence and density of iris strands or adhesions in the anterior chamber angle and the presence or absence of increased intraocular pressure. (9) This would suggest that the pathogenesis of the increased outflow resistance is related to some other factor and that the iris strands and adhesions may only represent a rough marker of an abnormal anterior chamber angle. Thirdly, the concept of the development of the angle of the anterior chamber by a process of "active cleavage and relative growth rather than by atrophy and resorption of mesodermal tissue" (3) has not been confirmed by other authors. (6, 11) Thus, defective anterior chamber cleavage probably does not represent a basis for the pathogenesis of this group of congenital and developmental anomalies. Finally, the association of this group of ocular anomalies with a variety of other systemic signs such as craniofacial and dental malformations (maxillary hypoplasia, microdontia, and anodontia), middle ear deafness, and malformations of the limbs and spine are difficult to explain in view of their apparently diverse embryologic origins. In fact, Cross and Maumanee may have had this in mind when they referred to some of these abnormalities as "mesoectodermal dysgenesis." (4)

The purpose of this paper is to review recent information on the development of the anterior chamber angle and associated structures and to present a new hypothesis to explain this group of clinical conditions.

A 23-month-old patient presenting the typical characteristics of Peter's anomaly (congenital corneal opacity with anterior synechiae to the opacity, iris adhesions to the trabecular meshwork, and increased intraocular pressure) underwent a trabeculectomy followed by a corneal transplantation. The tissue from these two operations was examined by light and electron microscopy. (7) Two findings were especially noteworthy. First, the corneal endothelium was not interrupted except at the area of the iris adhesion to the corneal opacity. However, the endothelial cells were abnormal in that they were extremely thin. Descemet's membrane was poorly defined, embryonal in appearance, being thin with a loosely packed basal lamina substance in which fine filaments and abundant electron-lucent collagen fibrils were intermingled. In the region of the iridocorneal adhesions, two layers of poorly defined Descemet's membrane were seen in loose connective tissue. The endothelial cells lining the trabecular beams of the meshwork contained phagocytosed pigment granules, and there was abundant wide-banded collagen fibrils with a periodicity of 1000 Å. Iris adhesions to the trabecular meshwork were confirmed histologically. By comparison, Schlemm's canal was lined with normal endothelial cells. The coexistence of abnormal corneal endothelial and trabecular endothelial cells to explain the corneal pathology and the accompanying glaucoma was confirmed in a second case seen more recently. This was a 35-year-old white woman who had slightly decreased vision in the right eye for as long as she could remember. When examined, vision in the right eye was 20/40 and in the left eye, 20/20. There was mild but definite nasal displacement of the pupils with a more prominent pupillary ruff temporally. Slit-lamp examination of the right cornea revealed mild stromal edema and linear opacities in Descemet's membrane as well as irregular thickening of the posterior corneal surface. The anterior iris stroma appeared thinned, but there was no transillumination. On gonioscopy, numerous rounded iris adhesions to the trabecular meshwork were noted. The intraocular pressure was 45 mm Hg on maximal medical therapy and a Bjerrum scotoma to the 14e was present. The optic nervehead showed an enlarged cup as compared to the fellow eye, but a normal flat pink rim was present. The left eye was normal, excepting the ectopic pupil and the presence of iris adhesions in the angle. The diagnosis was Rieger's anomaly with a corneal endothelial dystrophy. A trabeculectomy was performed and again the corneal endothelial cells and Descemet's membrane were abnormal, while a Descemet's-like membrane extended onto the trabecular meshwork. In addition, iris adhesions were confirmed.

During the past 30 years, there has been a sustained embryologic interest in the ontogeny of cells derived from the embryonic neural crest. The neural crest forms from the dorsal margin of the neural tube about the time of closure of the neural tube. The cells at this site undergo rapid division and begin to migrate extensively, playing an essential role in forming, among other things, certain spinal and cranial sensory ganglia, autonomic neurons, some pigment cells, odontoblasts, and some cephalic dermal bones. (12)

Recently, the migratory pattern of neural crest cells has been investigated by the use of a new cell marker system that consists of a large mass of chromatin found in the nuclei of cells of the Japanese quail. (8) This is in contrast to the rather diffuse chromatin pattern found in the cells of chick embryos that served as hosts for grafts of quail embryonic tissues. Since the quail chromatin replicates with each cell division and does not become diluted, the migration of these cells can be followed and their eventual location can be determined. The experiment consisted of transplanting naturally labeled quail neural crest cells into the neural crest region of a stage 35 chick embryo. Of particular interest to this discussion was the appearance of the quail neural crest cells in corneal stroma and endothelium, sclera, choroid, and the melanophores of the iris stroma. (5) More recently, it has been shown that the trabecular endothelial cells and the iris stroma (exclusive of muscle) are also derived from neural crest cells. On the other hand, the endothelial cells lining Schlemm's canal are formed from vascular mesoderm as is the blood vessel endothelium in general (JOHNSTON, personal communication). In addition, it is now clear that structures that often are involved in association with this group of anomalies of the cornea, iris and anterior chamber are also of neural crest origin. For instance, the bones of the face and portions of the floor of the cranial fossae as well as the dental papilla (odontoblasts) are derived from neural crest. Neural crest cells in the inner ear are apparently concerned with the regulation of inner ear fluid. (5) Finally, neural crest cell migration plays roles in the development of smooth and striated muscle, cartilige and bone, the meninges, and a variety of endocrine glands, thus helping to explain the association of craniofacial and dental malformations, middle ear deafness, and malformations of the upper spine with this group of ocular anomalies. (5)

Developmental anomalies of the anterior chamber associated with glaucoma may be best viewed in terms of problems of neural crest cell migration or perhaps a defective terminal induction of a particular structure from the neural crest cells. Abnormalities in the migration or terminal induction of corneal stroma may lead to a spectrum of corneal opacities as well as abnormalities in normal gwoth (megalocornea, microcornea). Defects in the corneal endothelium may result in defective Descemet's membrane and difficulty with appropriate corneal deturgescence as well as the clinical picture of an endothelial dystrophy. Such abnormal cells may also be inordinately "sticky", contributing to the formation of iridocorneal adhesions. The partial or complete absence of iris stromal tissue probably has profound secondary effect on the development and differentiation of the underlying pigmented and nonpigmented epithelium, leading to a number of pupil abnormalities (corectopia, dyscoria, iridotasis, slit pupil, ectropion of the pigmented epithelium) as well as additional induced defects in the pigmented epithelium (pseudopolycoria, atypical coloboma, or partial aniridia). If the defect in the iris stroma is severe enough to interfere with the development of adjacent structures such as the zonule and lens, ectopia lentis and anterior polar cataract may result.

With abnormalities of migration or terminal induction of the trabecular endothelial cells, problems in the maintenance of normal outflow resistance may result in elevated intraocular pressure. (5) This is not necessarily correlated with the amount or character of the iris strands or adhesions to the cornea or trabecular meshwork. Since so little is known about the function of the trabecular endothelial cell, further speculation must remain in abeyance. Finally, one need not invoke embryologic involvement other than the neural crest cell to explain the wide variety of associated systemic abnormalities.

Summary

The group of congenital and development anomalies of the anterior chamber associated with increased intraocular pressure has been difficult to interpret from an embryologic perspective that would take into account the ocular defects as well as associated systemic abnormalities. A new hypothesis is presented that suggests that the ocular and systemic defects can be explained by abnormalities in migration or terminal induction of neural crest cells. These cells represent the initial population that differentiates into the diversity of cell types that appear to be involved in both the ocular and systemic manifestation of this group of anterior chamber anomalies.

References

(1) Alkemade, P.P.H.: Dysgenesis mesodermalis of the iris and the cornea. Assen (Netherlands): Royal Van Gorcum 1969

(2) Allen, L.; Burian, H.M.; Braley, A.E.: A new concept of the development of the anterior chamber angle. Arch. Ophthalmol. 53, 783-798 (1955)

(3) Burian, H.M.; Braley, A.E.; Allen, L.: External and gonioscopic visibility of the ring of Schwalbe and the trabecular zone. Trans. Am. Ophthalmol. Soc. 51, 389-428 (1966)

(4) Cross, H.E.; Maumanee, A.E.: Progressive spontaneous dissolution of the iris. Surv. Ophthalmol. 18, 186-199 (1973)

(5) Johnston, M.C.; Bhakdinaronk, A.; Reid, Y.C.: An expanded role for the neural crest in oral and pharyngeal development. In: 4 Symposium on Oral Sensation and Perception, pp. 37-52. Washington (D.C.): U. S. Government Printing Office 1974

(6) Kupfer, C.: A note on the development of the anterior chamber angle. Invest. Ophthalmol. 8, 69-74 (1969)

(7) Kupfer, C.; Kuwabara, T.; Stark, W.J.: The histropathology of Peter's anomaly. Am. J. Ophthalmol. 80, 653-660 (1975)

(8) Le Doverin, N.: A biological cell labelling technique and its use in experimental embryology. Dev. Biol. 30, 217-22 (1973)

(9) Pearce, W.G.; Kerr, C.B.: Inherited variations in Rieger's malformation. B. J. Ophthalmol. 49, 530-537 (1965)

(10) Reese, A.B.; Ellsworth, R.M.: The anterior chamber cleavage syndrome. Arch. Ophthalmol. 75, 307-318 (1966)

(11) Smelser, G.K.; Ozanics, V.: The development of the trabecular meshwork in primate eyes. Am. J. Ophthalmol. 71, 366-385 (1971)

Results of Goniotomy and Trabeculotomy as the Initial Surgical Procedure in the Treatment of Congential Glaucoma

Celso Antonio de Carvalho, Alberto Jorge Betinjane, Mario Luiz Camargo

Rua Prof. Artur Ramos, 96 8º and., São Paulo - 01454, Brasil

Since 1968, we have been studying patients with congenital glaucoma according to the classification of gonioscopic features proposed by BUSACCA and CARVALHO (1,2). Three gonioscopic pictures have been considered: persistence, metaplasia, and aplasia of the reticular system of the pectinate ligament, depending on the intensity of the dysplasic process.

This approach to the study of congenital glaucoma has proved to be of special interest, mainly in relation to the most adequate surgical procedure to be adopted. We have thus seen (3) that, in general, among our patients, nearly 54 % present a preoperative gonioscopic picture of persistence of the pectinate ligament (65 % bilateral and 35% unilateral); 20 % show aplasia of that system (98 % bilateral); 7 % show metaplasia of that system (54 % bilateral and 46 % unilateral); and the remaining 19 % present conditions of corneal transparency that make it impossible to accurately assess the degree of mesodermic displasia that affected the anatomic elements constituting the chamber sinus.

There is no general agreement on the real existence of metaplasia of the reticular system, which we have been trying to characterize according to what we have previously described (1,2). In our experience, though a rare event, it undoubtedly exists as it has already been histologically demonstrated (4).

On the other hand, due to their socioeconomic status, many of our patients come to us when the disease has reached a very advanced stage and when it is absolutely impossible to obtain precise preoperative gonioscopic information on the nature of the chamber sinus anomaly. We have labeled them "impossible gonioscopy."

This experience led us to the study of the effectiveness of goniotomy (Worst's technique) and of trabeculotomy (Mackensen's technique) in a group of patients who have returned for evaluation of post-operative results and who had a follow-up period of not less than 3 years.

Method

Two hundred ninety-four eyes of 181 patients were studied: 57.45 % (104 patients) had persistence, 8.28 % (15 patients) metaplasia, 13.8 % (25 patients) aplasia of the reticular system, and 20.4 % (37 patients) were classified as impossible gonioscopy in the preoperative period. Regarding age, race, and sex, the 181 patients were distributed as shown in Table 1.

Table 1.

Gonioscopic pictures	Race			Sex		Age(years)			
	W	B	Y	Masc	Fem	0-1	1-2	2-5	5-10
Persistence	94	9	1	58	46	73	4	10	17
Metaplasia	15	-	-	6	9	13	2	-	-
Aplasia	24	-	1	16	9	16	3	4	2
Impossible	35	2	-	25	12	25	5	6	1

W, white; B, Black; Y, Yellow; Masc, = masculine; Fem, = feminine

On admission, after preliminary anamnesis, patients were submitted to ocular examination under sedation, obtained either by oral Nembutal (10 mg/kg of body weight), inhalation of Pentrane (depending on the body weight of the child), or topical anesthesia of the cornea with 0.5 % tetracaine, if they were old enough to allow satisfactory examination conditions.

The routine of ocular examination included applanation tonometry (Draeger tonometer), measurement of the horizontal corneal diameter with compasses, biomicroscopy of the cornea, anterior chamber, iris, and lens, ophthalmoscopy, and, finally the gonioscopic study of the anterior chamber periphery with Goldmann's contact lens.

Postoperative examinations were repeated 1, 3, 9, and 12 months after surgery, and every 6 months thereafter, following the same criteria used for the initial examination. This routine has been satisfactory since we can get excellent sedation with oral Nembutal in patients up to 11 kg of body weight. It is adequate for our working conditions since we cannot rely on general anesthesia for all initial examinations, which are always performed before the general anesthesia needed for the planned surgical procedure.

The maintenance of postoperative intraocular pressure below 20 mm Hg is considered a satisfactory surgical result, provided the intolerance to light has disappeared and the corneal diameter does not show siginificant changes during the follow-up period.

Results and Discussion

The 294 eyes were distributed to correlate the gonioscopic picture, the mean intraocular pressure before surgery and after goniotomy or trabeculotomy, and the mean horizontal corneal diameter. These data are presented in Tables 2 - 5 for every group of eyes included in the different gonioscopic situations. As Table 2 indicates, the percentage of surgical successes and failures with goniotomy and trabeculotomy in persistence was similar, i.e. 77.17 % and 74.4 %, respectively.

Table 2. Persistence of the reticular system of the pectinate ligament (163 eyes)

	No. of eyes	Final result	No. of eyes	Corneal diameters	Intraocular pressure (before)	Intraocular pressure (after)	Percentual result
Goniotomy	92	Suc	71	13.14 ± 0.84	28.16 ± 6.57	12.27 ± 3.16	77.17 %
		Unsuc	21	14.16 ± 0.91	26.79 ± 4.8	28.25 ± 4.4	22.82 %
Trabeculotomy	71	Suc	53	13.13 ± 1.03	27.7 ± 9.6	12.6 ± 4.4	74.4 %
		Unsuc	18	14.0 ± 1.1	32.9 ± 7.2	30.2 ± 7.9	25.35 %

Suc, = successful; Unsuc, = unsuccessful

As far as metaplasia is concerned, all of the eyes included in the present study were submitted to goniotomy, since the conditions were favorable to the performance of that technique. Twenty-one of the eyes with metaplasia were submitted to goniotomy: 15 eyes (71.4 %) presented successful results and six eyes (28.57 %) unsuccessful results (Table 3).

Table 3. Metaplasia of the reticular system of the pectinate ligament (21 eyes)

	No. of eyes	Final result	No. of eyes	Corneal diameters	Intraocular pressure (before)	Intraocular pressure (After)	Percentual result
Goniotomy	21	Suc.	15	13.3 ± 1.03	24.9 ± 4.4	10.9 ± 1.6	71.42 %
		Unsuc	6	13.1 ± 0.5	21.9 ± 2.5	27.3 ± 6.0	28.57 %

Suc, = successful; Unsuc, = unsuccessful

In the 45 eyes with aplasia of the reticular system (Table 4), the initial examination showed 16 eyes with conditions of corneal transparency favorable to the performance of goniotomy. Of these 16 eyes, we obtained surgical success in only three eyes (18.7 %). On the other hand, trabeculotomy was performed as the first surgical procedure on 29 eyes: successfully on 21 eyes (72.4 %) and unsuccessfully on eight eyes (27.6 %).

Table 4. Aplasia of the reticular system of the pectinate ligament (45 eyes)

	No. of eyes	Final result	No. of eyes	Corneal diameters	Intraocular pressure (before)	Intraocular Pressure (after)	Percentual result
Goniotomy	16	Suc.	3	13.0 ± 0.5	32.7 ± 3.74	14.0 ± 0.78	18.7 %
		Unsuc	13	12.6 ± 1.67	35.8 ± 5.09	30.6 ± 3.35	81.3 %
Trabeculotomy	29	Suc	21	13.3 ± 0.9	27.5 ± 5.0	14.0 ± 2.72	72.4 %
		Unsuc	8	14.3 ± 0.84	29.6 ± 7.41	26.7 ± 5.19	27.6 %

Suc, = successful; Unsuc, = unsuccessful

The eyes that did not present any conditions for the performance of controlled goniotomy under surgical microscopy due to poor corneal conditions were submitted to trabeculotomy. Of 65 eyes (Table 5), we achieved surgical success in 44 eyes (67.6%). It is evident that this group corresponds to eyes of poor surgical prognosis; however, it corresponds in our socioeconomic group to nearly 20 % of the diagnosis of congenital glaucoma. We thus notice that trabeculotomy allows for good results also in those eyes where the performance of goniotomy is practically impossible.

Table 5. Impossible gonioscopy (65 eyes)

	No. of eyes	Final result	No. of eyes	Corneal diameters	Intraocular pressure (before)	Intraocular pressure (after)	Percentual result
Trabeculotomy	65	Suc	44	13.7 ± 1.07	28.4 ± 8.36	13.1 ± 4.5	67.6 %
		Unsuc	21	14.3 ± 1.07	32.45 ± 6.92	26.2 ± 8.1	32.3 %

Suc, = successful; Unsuc, = unsuccessful

Considering the surgical results in the different groups of eyes classified according to the gonioscopic features, we could observe that the group of eyes with persistence presents almost equivalent results with goniotomy and trabeculotomy; on the other hand, the aplasia group presented a clearly greater success with trabeculotomy (72.4 %) as compared to the success obtained with goniotomy (28.57 %). If we consider the unfeasibility of goniotomy in the group of impossible gonioscopy, the results achieved through trabeculotomy may be deemed satisfactory (67.7 % success in the eyes submitted to surgery).

Although goniotomy is an excellent surgical technique to section the trabeculae of the persistent reticular system of the pectinate ligament, it requires ideal conditions of corneal transparency necessary not only to the performance of the correct surgical act under direct visualization and under microscopy but also to the preoperative diagnosis of the mesodermic displasia that attains the chamber sinus. On the other hand, goniotomy is not indicated as a surgical procedure for cases of aplasia of the reticular system , since only 18.7 % successful results were obtained. It seems evident, therefore, that the preoperative gonioscopic study presents practical and useful information as to the best surgical procedure to be adopted for any given case of congenital glaucoma.

Concerning the importance of the corneal diameter on the surgical results, we have statistically evaluated the significance of the difference of two means, comparing the group of eyes operated by goniotomy to those operated by trabeculotomy, with and without success. Although the values of the mean corneal diameters of eyes operated with success were often lower than those operated without success, such differences were not statistically significant for the Student - test and for a 5 % probability.

From this study, we gather that trabeculotomy, when compared to goniotomy, is the surgical procedure that offers better and wider possibilities for the treatment of congenital glaucoma, whatever the conditions of corneal transparency or the nature of the anomaly of the chamber sinusis.

For the sake of comparison, we thought it useful to present some aspects of the normal contralateral eye of 46 patients with unilateral congenital glaucoma who were included in this study. We have found a mean corneal diameter of 11.45 ± 0.81 mm Hg and a mean intraocular pressure under oral Nembutal of 11.7 ± 2.42 mm Hg in patients who were less than 12 months old. In that same group of eyes, we noticed wide corneal limubs in all of the eyes and a persistence of pectinate trabeculae of variable degree in 92 % of the eyes that were considered normal.

Summary

From the gonioscopic point of view, 294 eyes of 181 congenital glaucoma patients were studied in the preoperative stage and submitted to goniotomy or trabeculotomy as the first surgical procedure. The percentual frequency of good operative results was statistically studied to evaluate the importance of the corneal diameter in the success of the surgical result. No statistical significance was established in relation to the corneal diameter when goniotomy or trabeculotomy were considered. The importance of the gonioscopic study of the periphery of the anterior chamber in the preoperative stage is stressed in relation to the indication of the most adequate surgical procedure (goniotomy or trabeculotomy) to be adopted.

References

(1) Busacca, A.; Carvalho, C.A.: La morphogénèse du sinus camérulaire étudie par la gonioscopie. Ann. Oculist. 201, 400-430 (1968)

(2) Busacca, A.; Carvalho, C.A.: La gonioscopie du glaucome congénital Ann. Oculist. 201, 887-919 (1968)

(3) Carvalho, C.A.; Betinjane, A.J.; Camargo, M.L.: Some features of the congenital glaucoma. Rev. Bras. Oftalmol. (in press) (1978)

(4) Campos, F.C.: Desarrollo y anomalias del angulo camerular del ojo. Ph. D. Thesis, University of Lima (Peru) 1972

Congenital Glaucoma: Light and Scanning Electron Microscopy of Trabeculectomy Specimens

Roberto Sampaolesi, Jorge O. Zarate, Rafael Caruso

University of Salvador, Department of Ophthalmology,
Paraná 1239-1°, Buenos Aires, Argentina

Until 1968, we treated congenital glaucoma with goniotomy according to Barkan's technique. With this method, we achieved favorable results in 65 % of the cases (in some after three goniotomies). Since 1969, we consider trabeculotomy according to Harms' technique the surgical procedure of choice in congenital glaucoma. Our first results were published in 1972 (13). At present we have been able to control the intraocular pressure in 96 % of our cases (120 cases followed from 1 - 9 years).

Nevertheless, in a group of cases, trabeculotomy is ineffective in controling intraocular pressure within its normal levels (3,11,14) for children from birth to 3 years of age. In these cases, the horizontal diameter of the cornea is 13.5 mm, or larger, Descemet's membrane shows the characteristic tears, and the axial length of the eye is increased (determined by echometry). They are, in fact, congenital glaucomas of advanced evolution that undergo surgical treatment too late. In these cases, we performed a combined technique of trabeculotomy and trabeculectomy (strictly speaking: partial sinusectomy or goniectomy).

The purpose of this paper is to describe the trabeculectomy specimens obtained from these children, studied with light and scanning electron microscopy.

Material (Table 1)

The trabeculectomy specimens were obtained from: two 4-month-old infants, two 6-month-old infants, one 2-year-old child and two 3-year old children (seven specimens). We also studied trabeculectomy specimens from late congenital glaucoma of long evolution: one 7-year-old child, one 10-year-old child, one 12-year-old child, and one 15-year-old child (four specimens). Finally, we studied two specimens, one from a 33-year-old adult with pigmentary glaucoma and one from a 32-year-old adult with late congenital glaucoma (two specimens). In all, 13 trabeculectomy specimens have been analyzed.

Table 1.

Case	Age	Sex	IOP		Corneal diameter		Descemet tears		Ecometry			
									TL	V	TL	V
			OD	OS	OD	OS	OD	OS	OD		OS	
1	4 mo	♂	30	35	13	12.2	+	+	22.61	14.55	22.85	14.55
2	4 mo	♀	10	33	12	14	-	+	22.31	14.32	23.53	15.32
3	6 mo	♂	20	18	14.5	14.5	+	+	23.83	15.09	23.59	15.32
4	6 mo	♂	30	30	14	13.5	+	+	24.14	15.47	23.76	14.94
5	2 yr	♀	36	18	13.5	12	+	-	24.04	16.09	21.50	13.32
6	3 yr	♂	29	26	13.5	13.5	+	+	23.52	15.17	23.37	15.32
7	3 yr	♂	34	10	14	12	+	N	28.09	19.15	21.78	14.02
8	10 yr	♂	34	31	14	14.5	-	-	28.54	19.92	28.36	19.53
9	12 yr	♂	25	24	14	14	-	-	24.81	16.24	24.01	16.24
10	7 yr	♂	34	13			-	-	23.23		23.08	
11	14 yr	♂	32	52	12	12						
12	33 yr	♂	38	32	12	12	-	-				
13	32 yr	♀	26	16	12	12	-	-				

IOP, intraocular pressure; OD, oculus dexter; OS, oculus sinister; TL, total

Method

Procurement of the trabeculectomy specimens. We consider that meticulous surgical technique and careful manipulation of the piece of trabecular meshwork during its excision are very important. Transillumination, as described by MINSKY, is essential to place the incision at the level of the corneal endothelium immediately beyond Schwalbe's ring. This technique allows us to section the cornea in the area of light, at 1 mm from the limit of light and darkness. After dissection of a limbus-based scleral flap, Minsky's maneuver allows us to place the first incision parallel to the limbus. We section only half the thickness of the cornea. Before opening the anterior chamber, we mark the lateral incisions and section half the thickness of the scleral wall. After opening the anterior chamber, we complete the first incision with an angled Vannas scissors (Storz). With the same instrument, we complete the lateral incisions perpendicular to the limbus. The trabeculectomy piece is gently grasped with fine-toothed microsurgical forceps (Grieshaber) by the external half of its thickness to avoid damaging the delicate structure of the meshwork. The chamber angle is then exposed to the surgeon's eye, and the final incision is performed with Vannas scissors between the scleral spur and the ciliary band.

The specimens for light microscopy were embedded in paraffin and stained with the following techniques: hematoxylin-eosin stain, Masson trichrome stain, PAS stain, and the Gomori and Del Río Hortega method for reticulin.

Gonioscopy mesodermal remnants OD	Gonioscopy mesodermal remnants OS	Pathology mesodermal remnants Diffuse	Ligamentous	cM displaced	Post op IOP	Follow-up	Pupillary displacem. OD	Pupillary displacem. OS
Diffuse lig.	Diffuse lig.	x	-	x	10 10	3 yr	-	-
-	-	-	-	-	10 8	2 mo	-	-
Diffuse Aplasia	Diffuse Aplasia	x	x	-	10 11	3 yr	-	-
Diffuse lig.	Diffuse lig.	x	x	x	8 8	7 mo	+	+
Diffuse	-	x	-	-	10 12	2 yr	+	-
Diffuse		x	-	x	9 9	1 yr	-	+
Diffuse		x	-	-	11 10	16 mo	-	-
Diffuse Aplasia		x (dense)	-	-	16 14	14 mo	-	-
Diffuse?	Aplasia	x?	-	-	18 18	1 yr	-	-
		-	x	-	12 13	2 yr	-	-
		x		x	17 18	2 yr	-	-
Diffuse Ligament.	Diffuse Ligament.		x		18 18	4 yr	-	-
Diffuse Ligament.	Diffuse Ligament.	x	x		14 15	2 yr	-	-

length; V, vitreas; cM, ciliary muscle

The specimens for scanning electron microscopy (SEM) were immediately fixed by immersion in 2.5% glutaraldehyde in 0.1 M Millonig's phosphate buffer with glucose, pH 7.4 for about 24 h. After being rinsed in isotonic buffer for 15 min, the specimen is postfixed in 1% osmium tetroxide in Millonig's phosphate buffer with glucose, pH 7.4 for 2 h. Thereafter, the sample is dehydrated in graded acetone solutions and dried by the critical point method in fluid CO_2 with a Sorvall Critical Point Drying System. This method allows the substitution of acetone by carbon dioxide in a high-pressure chamber. Once dried, the trabeculectomy piece is mounted on a specimen holder, with the trabecular meshwork facing upward, and coated with a thin layer of carbon and gold palladium in a Jeol vacuum-coating unit. The piece is examined in a JSM-U 3 scanning electron microscope.

Mesodermal Remnants in the Chamber Angle

We find that a precise definition of the nature and appearance of the mesodermal remnants is essential for the interpretation of the gonioscopic and histopathologic findings. The mesodermal tissue found in the first stages of development in the chamber angle can suffer a number of alterations in its differentiation process. The morphologic expression of this differentiation is the resorption of the pre-existent mesodermal tissue (6,7,9,17). When this differentiation (resorption) process is altered, there is a persistence of undifferentiated mesodermal tissue (10,15). Different authors have named this alteration: mesodermal remnants, pectinate ligament, and pathologic uveal meshwork.

Barkan's membrane can be identified in gonioscopy by its translucent appearance. We can see through it, as if in a haze, the mesodermal remnants of the chamber angle. At times, it shows thinner areas with holes through which these remnants can be seen directly. The papers by HANSSON and JERNDAL (5) and SMELSER and OZANICS (17) give histologic support to its existence: nevertheless, it is rarely found in conventional sections. We propose the following classification of these mesodermal remnants according to morphologic criteria.

Normal Remnants: Iris Processes

Iris processes consist of a central axis of collagen and a lesser number of reticulin fibres with fibroblasts enveloped by numerous melanocytes. In other words, their structure is identical to that of the superficial mesodermal layer of the iris (Fig.1). Iris processes run from the inner wall of the chamber angle (iris) to its outer wall (sclera cornea). The iridic end of the processes never extends beyond the base of the last circular fold of the iris, that is to say, they never start from the iris root. Their corneoscleral end may reach different heights at the outer wall of the chamber angle (corneoscleral meshwork: scleral spur, trabecular meshwork at the level of Schlemm's canal or Schwalbe's ring), but they never extend beyond the latter.

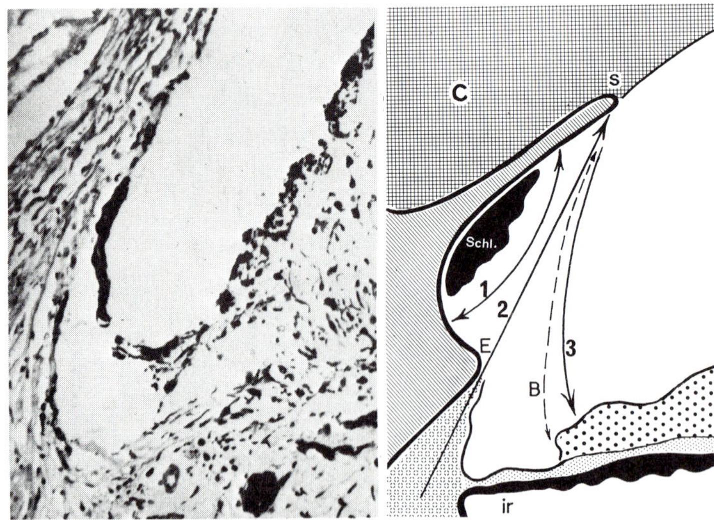

Fig.1 (a) Normal iris process. (b) ir, iris root; S, Schwalbe's line; E, scleral spur; Schl, Schlemm's canal; 1, corneoscleral meshwork; 2, ciliary muscle tendon; 3, iris process; B, site of Barkan's membrane

Pathologic Remnants

Diffuse mesodermal remnants are the most frequently observed remnants of the chamber angle in our congenital glaucoma specimens (Table 1). In gonioscopy, it appears as a band of tissue that can be seen in the whole chamber angle circumference and covers the structure of the outer chamber angle wall to a lesser or greater extent (ciliary body band, scleral spur, trabecular meshwork). The gonioscopic appearance of congenital glaucoma is usually the absence (no visibility) of the ciliary body band, because it is covered by the mesodermal remnants and looks like a high insertion of the iris in the corneoscleral wall (Fig. 2). In light microscopy sections, it appears as a lax fibrilar meshwork made up of reticular and, to a lesser degree, collagen fibers, with endothelial cells and, occasionally, with fine granular pigments. It extends as a net or mesh in the chamber angle from the iris root to Schwalbe's ring.

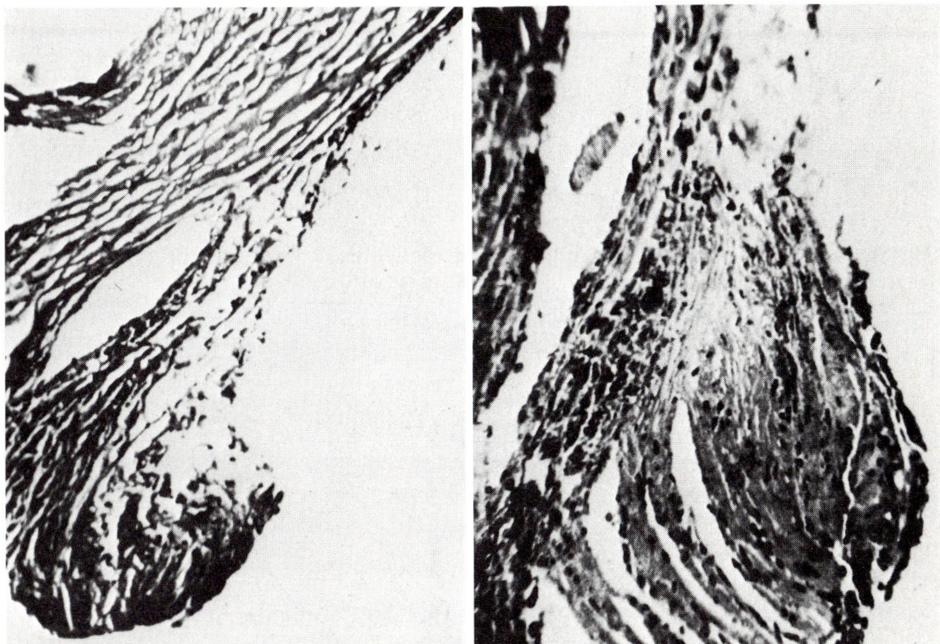

Fig. 2 (a) Pathologic remnants: ligamentous, with normal position of the ciliary muscle. (b) Pathologic remnants: ligamentous, displaced ciliary muscle

Ligamentous mesodermal remnants are less frequently found in our cases. They can be observed in histologic sections, although they are not easily evidenced. They extend from the iris root (not from the last circular fold of the iris) to the outer wall of the chamber angle, rising no further than Schwalbe's ring, and consist of a fibrillar structure made up only of reticulin fibres with interfibrillar spaces and occasionally pigmented cells over the surface (Fig. 3).

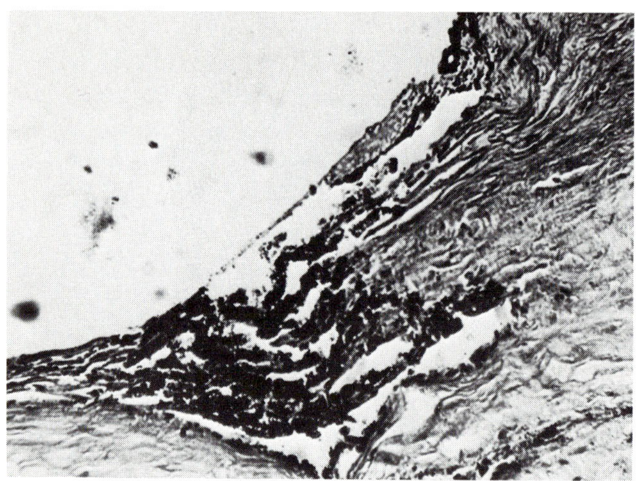

Fig.3. Pathologic remnants: ligamentous

Obviously, the borderline between normal and pathologic mesodermal remnants is not sharp, and there is an intermediate area that makes their gonioscopic interpretation difficult. Nevertheless, it is possible to classify these remnants as follows (based exclusively on morphologic criteria without prejudgment of the pathogenic significance of these structures in congenital glaucoma):

Mesodermal Tissue of the Chamber Angle	Normal	Corneoscleral meshwork Iris root Iris processes	Collagen and reticular
	Pathologic Remnants	Diffuse Ligamentous	Reticular and Collagen

The structures just described have been differentiated according to two criteria:

a) Topographic: (1) gonioscopy, (2) study and photography of the trabeculectomy specimens under slit-lamp or surgical microscope, and (3) appraisal of the position of the elements of the chamber angle in low power light microscopy.

b) Morphologic: according to the staining properties of different tissues, using the hematoxylin-eosin stain, PAS stain, Masson trichrome stain, and the Gomori and Del Rio Hortega technique for reticulin.

In a section of a trabeculectomy (partial sinusectomy) specimen stained with hematoxylin-eosin, both topographic and some morphologic criteria can be inferred. One limitation of this technique is that collagen cannot be differentiated from reticular structures. Thus, adequate techniques must be additionally employed. The PAS stain provides few further topographic details in these specimens, but it is useful to detect the amount of reticulin in mesodermal remnants. The Masson trichrome stain is particularly useful to ascertain with ease the position of the ciliary muscle and the scleral spur with a topographic criterium. In addition, collagen and reticular structures can be adequately differentiated: the trabecular meshwork stains blue and the diffuse and ligamentous mesodermal remnants stain pink. The silver

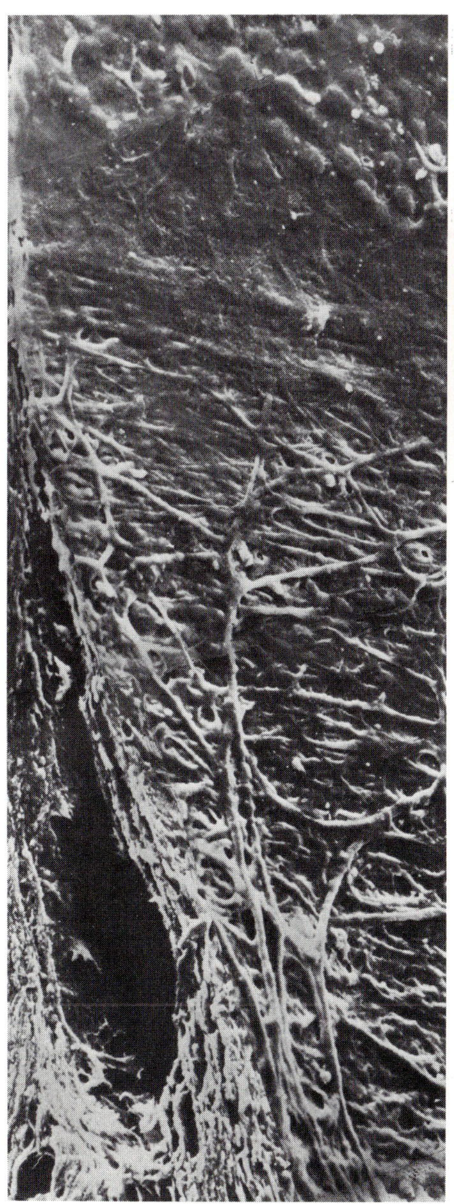

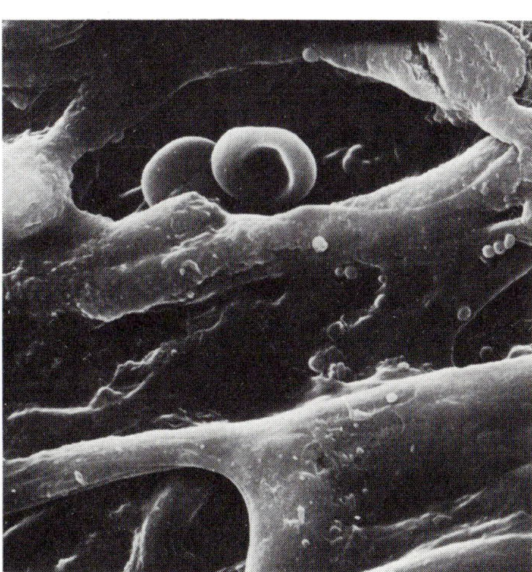

Fig. 4 (a) Scanning electron microscopy: normal trabecular meshwork (× 300). (b) Detail from Fig. 4a (× 300)

impregnation procedure for reticulin fibres allows us to appreciate the quantity of these fibers, a fact that may be overlooked using the other preceding methods.

Scanning Electron Microscopy

We have studied five specimens corresponding to case histories 3,4,7,8,9, and 13 (Table 1). In every case, we observed in the inner surface diffuse mesodermal remnants and some ligamentous mesodermal remnants in relief, formed by the

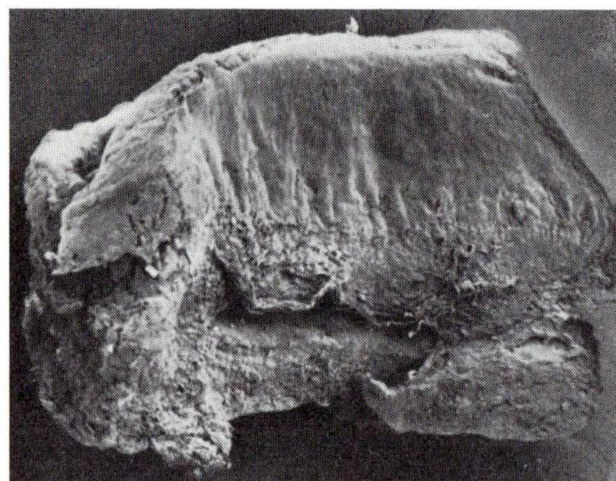

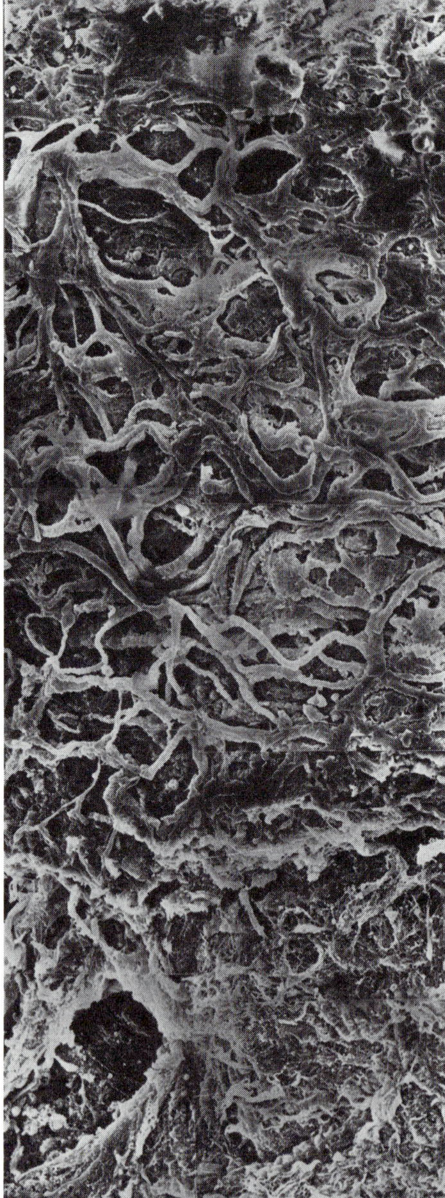

Fig.5 (a) Congenital glaucoma. Trabeculectomy specimen with Schlemm's canal opened with a trabeculotome. The trabeculotomy on the left of the specimen is incomplete to show that the trabeculotome opens the outer wall of Schlemm's canal (× 75). (b) Detail from Fig.5a. Trabecular meshwork (× 300)

tortuous and very thickened trabeculae. Between the latter, instead of intertrabecular spaces, we found membranes (endothelium?) occluding these spaces (Fig.6a, case 13). Only some small holes and pores are present, smaller then the diameter of red blood cells, which, therefore, are deformed and unable to pass through the meshwork (Fig.6b). For the sake of comparison, a normal trabecular meshwork is shown (Fig.4a) with red blood cells passing through freely (Fig.4b). Figure 5 (case 3) shows a trabeculectomy specimen of a 6-month-old infant with the same appearance. Both gonioscopy and scanning electron microscopy only allowed us to detect the presence of diffuse and ligamentous mesodermal remnants but gave us no evidence about the position of the ciliary muscle.

Light Microscopy

First group: analyzing the seven specimens belonging to infants and children from 4 months to 3 years of age (Table 1), diffuse mesodermal remnants could be found in six. Ligamentous mesodermal remnants were found only in two cases (case 4, 6-month-old infant, and case 3, 4-month-old infant). We remind the reader that it is difficult to evidence these remnants in histologic sections. In three cases (1,4, and 6), the ciliary muscle was displaced and reached up to the level of the middle Schlemm's canal (Fig.2).

The only case showing a trabecular specimen of normal appearance, without mesodermal remnants, was that of a 4-month-old infant to whom dexamethasone eye drops had been administered twice daily for 3 months. The histologic characteristics were identical to those of the two specimens of cortisonic glaucomas of the adult that we studied. These findings, and those of a case that could be proposed for discussion, emphasize the fact that in our trabecular specimens we were unable to find the histologic counterpart of the gonioscopic appearance of the aplasia of mesodermal remnants, called "aplasia of the pectinate ligament" by BUSACCA. Therefore, light microscopy, when compared with scanning electron microscopy, allows us a more precise study about the nature of pathologic mesodermal remnants and gives evidence about the position of the ciliary muscle. Nevertheless, scanning electron microscopy allows us to identify the membranes that occlude the intertrabecular spaces.

Second group: in case 10 (age 7) ligamentous mesodermal remnants were seen, and in case 11 (age 15) both diffuse mesodermal remnants and a displacement of the ciliary muscle were found. The topographic appearance of the specimen from case 8 (age 10) was that of a normal chamber angle, without mesodermal remnants but with a very dense trabecular meshwork. Nevertheless, the Gomori silver impregnation showed a large number of reticulin fibers, typically found in mesodermal remnants. This is possibly a congenital glaucoma of long evolution in which the structures that look like a dense trabecular meshwork may actually have a different origin (mesodermal remnants). In the specimen from case 9 (age 12), Schlemm's canal was divided into three parts, and inflammatory signs and angular synechias were seen. This case was classified as a secondary glaucoma due to these findings, even though the horizontal corneal diameter was enlarged.

Third group: in case 13 (late congenital glaucoma in a 32-year-old female patient), ligamentous mesodermal remnants were found. Figure 6 shows the scanning electron microphotography of this case. In case 12 (pigmentary glaucoma in a 33-year-

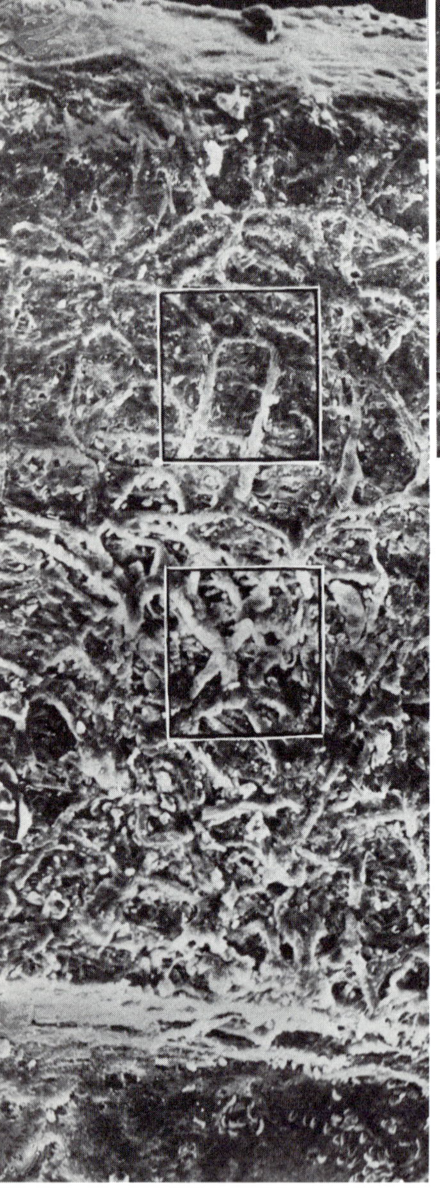

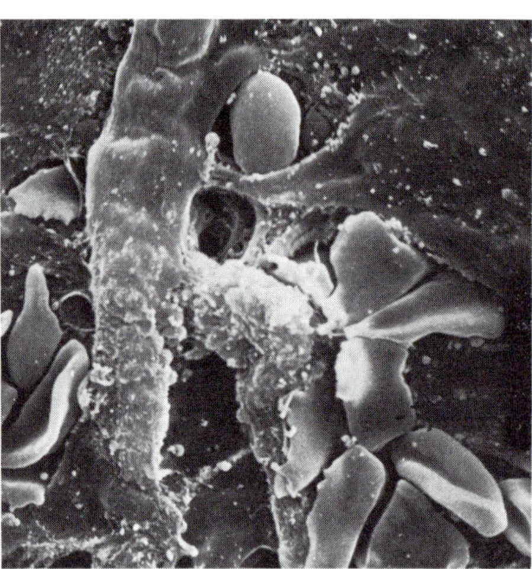

Fig.6 (a) Scanning electron microscopy: late congenital glaucoma (× 300). (b) Detail from Fig.6a (× 3000)

old male patient), Masson's trichrome stain shows the trabecular meshwork full of pigment granules as is usual in this syndrome. The most significant finding with this stain are ligamentous mesodermal remnants that are stained pink, in contrast to the normal trabecular meshwork that is stained blue (Fig. 3). These histologic features, when related to the clinical findings (atrophy of the pigmentary layer of the iris, trapezoidal anterior chamber, peripheral iridodonesis, a chamber angle depression in the inferior nasal quadrant, anterior vitreous detachment with a floating anterior hyaloid membrane, myopia, optic disk disversion etc.), relate this syndrome, also from the histologic standpoint, to the congenital glaucomas of late onset (8,12,16).

Clinical and Surgical Considerations

It can be ascertained from the data presented in Table 1 that, in addition to the features we have already described in these glaucomas, there is an increase in the axial length of the eye when measured by echometry. There is a precise correlation in the cases of unilateral glaucoma, in which this increase is only present in the affected eye. These measurements have been evaluated according to the GERNET and HOLLWICH curves for normal and glaucomatous eyes.

In all the cases described, the intraocular pressure reached a normal level postoperatively. The period of postoperative control ranges between 7 months and 3 years. A postoperative complication that we shall try to avoid in the future was seen in three cases of the first group of children, with ages between 4 months and 3 years. At the site of the trabeculectomy, even though a peripheral iridectomy was performed, a large angular synechia developed, leaving the trabeculectomy in communication with the posterior chamber. This synechia displaces the pupil upward, changing its shape into a vertical slit (cat's pupil). This complication can be avoided with a large peripheral iridectomy. It must be remembered that when only a trabeculotomy is performed three postoperative angular synechias are seen: one is central and trapezoidal in shape, and the others are lateral and triangular, but the pupila is never displaced (120 observations). Even though the central synechia is present, and the pigmentation sometimes reaches the corneal endothelium, there is no pupillary displacement.

Summary.

In a series of cases of advanced congenital glaucoma in infants and children from 4 months to 3 years of age (horizontal corneal diameter larger than 13.5 mm and axial length of the eye larger than normal, according to their age as measured by echometry), trabeculectomy had to be added to trabeculotomy as a combined surgical procedure to control the intraocular pressure. The study of the trabeculectomy specimen (partial goniectomy or sinusectomy) with light and scanning electron microscopy allowed us to draw to the following conclusions:

1) Pathologic mesodermal remnants are present in the chamber angle and appear in two different forms: diffuse mesodermal remnants and ligamentous mesodermal remnants in that order of frequency. 2) These pathologic mesodermal remnants contain more reticular than collagen fibers (stained with PAS, Masson, and Gomori); the contrary is valid for the trabecular meshwork, iris processes, etc. 3) The aplasia of this mesodermal tissue, as described by BUSACCA, which shows a distinct gonioscopic appearance, was not identified in our series. 4) In some cases of very long evolution that had been operated late, the only alteration found was a very dense trabecular meshwork. Only an impregnation method for reticulin fiber (Gomori) allowed us to determine that this meshwork is composed mainly by reticulin fibers, in contrast to the normal findings. This suggests that this structure is a different trabecular meshwork, made up of diffuse mesodermal remnants compressed by a high intraocular pressure of long standing. 5) In three cases of congenital glaucoma, besides the persistence of diffuse mesodermal remnants, the position of the ciliary muscle shows a forward displacement, its anterior wall reaching the level of the middle of Schlemm's canal. 6) The histopathologic study allowed us to modify our diagnosis of congenital glaucoma, notwithstanding the large corneal diameter in two cases: one cortisonic glaucoma and one secondary glaucoma. 7) In pigmentary glaucoma, we have found ligamentous mesodermal remnants with staining properties totally unlike those of the corneosclearl trabecular meshwork (Masson trichrome stain). 8) Scanning electron microscopy of congenital glaucoma specimens allowed us to identify thickened trabeculae with disappearance of the intertrabecular spaces, which are occluded by a membrane (endothelium?) that shows small pores that do not allow red blood cells to pass through them.

References

(1) Busacca, A.; Carvalho, C.A.: La morphologie du sinus camérulaire étudié par la gonioscopie. Ann. Oculist. (Paris) 201, 400-430 (1968)

(2) Busacca, A.; Carvalho, C.A.: La gonioscopie due glaucome congénital (I). Ann. Oculist. (Paris) 201, 887-919 (1968)

(3) Carvalho, C.A.; Calixto, N.: Semiologia do glaucoma congenito. XV Congresso Brasileiro de Oftalmologie. pp. 101-1974 (1969)

(4) Gernet, H.; Hollwich, F.: Oculometrie des kindlichen Glaukoms. Ber. Dtsch. Ophthal. Ges. 69, 341-348 (1969)

(5) Hansson, H.A.; Jerndal, T.: Scanning electron microscopic studies on the development of the iridocorneal angle in human eyes. Invest. Ophthalmal. 10, 252-265 (1971)

(6) Kupfer, C.: Gonioscopy in infants and children. Diagnostic procedures in pediatric opthalmology. Apt, L. (ed.), pp. 11-23. London: Churchill 1963

(7) Kupfer, C.: A note on the development of the anterior chamber angle. Invest. Ophthalmol. 8, 69-74 (1969)

(8) Malbran, J.: Le glaucome pigmentarie, se relations avec le glaucoma congénital. Probl. act. Ophthal. 1, pp. 132-146 (1957)

(9) Mann, L.C.: The development of the human eye. Cambridge Univ. Press: 1928. 2nd ed. London 1949

(10) Maumennee, A.: Further observations on the pathognesis of congenital glaucoma. Trans. Am. Ophthalmol. 60, 40 (1962)

(11) Radthke, N.; Cohan, B.: Intraocular pressure measurement in the newborn. Am. J. Ophthalmol. 78, 501-504 (1974)

(12) Sampaolesi, R.:Le glaucome dit pigmentaire. Son rapport avec le glaucome congénital. Bull. Soc. Ophthalmol. Fr. 80, 434-463 (1968)

(13) Sampaolesi, R.: Die Trabeculotomie als erste Operation fürs kongenitale Glaukom, bei Kindern bis zum ersten Lebensjahr. Ber. Dtsch. Ophthalmol. Ges. 71, 358-371 (1972)

(14) Sampaolesi, R.; Reca, R.; Carro, A.; Armando, A.: Normaler intraocularer Druck bei Kindern bis zu 5 Jahren mit und ohne Allgemeinnarkose. Seine Wichtigkeit für die Frühdiagnose des angeborenen Glaukoms. Glaukom Symposium, Würzburg 1974. pp. 278-289 Stuttgart: Enke 1976

(15) Seefelder, R.; Wolfrum: Zur Entwicklung der vorderen Kammer und des Kammerwinkels beim Menschen nebst Bemerkungen über ihre Entstehung bei Tieren. Albrecht von Graefes Arch. Klin Ophthalmol. 63, 430-451 (1906)

(16) Shaffer, R.N.; Weiss, D.I.: Congenital and pediatric glaucomas. St. Louis: Mosby 1970

(17) Smelser, G.K.; Ozanics, V.: The development of the trabecular meshwork in primate eye. Am. J. Ophthalmol. 71, 366-385 (1971)

Otto Barkan and the Pathophysiology of Primary Congenital (Infantile) Glaucoma

Robert N. Shaffer

University of California, Glaucoma Clinic A 775, San Francisco, Cal. 94143, USA

It has been 40 years since Otto BARKAN first tried goniotomy for control of infantile glaucoma. It has been 36 years since his first paper appeared describing the success of the operation. (1) His technique and his gonioscopic observations of the chamber angle remain unchallenged today. Gonioscopically, BARKAN noted the hypoplastic iris stroma that expose the peripheral pigment layer in an arcade-like fashion. The iris inserted higher than usual into a translucent, gelatinous angle tissue whose surface looked like stippled cellophane. He thought that this tissue was a fetal mesodermal reticulum filling an otherwise normal angle. He believed that goniotomy restored normal drainage by clearing away this reticulum. We are not far from that belief today.

The earliest report of the pathology of early congenital glaucoma was by SEEFELDER in 1906. (11) His findings were confirmed and elaborated by MAUMENEE in 1958 and 1962. (6, 7, 12) The gonioscopic appearance is caused by a hypoplasia of the iris. The peripheral iris inserts directly into the trabecular surface. The chamber angle is fetal in type, like a fetus of 7 - 8 months of gestation. There is a rudimentary development of the scleral spur with Schlemm's canal posterior to the iris attachment. A large part of the longitudinal muscles insert directly into the thick persistent uveal meshwork. It is this thick meshwork with its shagreened membranous surface that produces the gelatinous appearance described by Barkan. Worst is convinced that the resistance to outflow is at this surface, which he calls "Barkan's membrane." (17) Most pathologists, including MAUMENEE, tend to reject this hypothesis because a convincing surface membrane is not always seen in microscopic sections.

SAMPAOLESI makes a distinction between eyes with a "pectinate ligament" and those with a Barkan membrane. (11) We would call his pectinate ligament uveal meshwork, believing that the Barkan membrane is present as the inner layer of the meshwork in all eyes. SAMPAOLESI also distinguishes a type of congenital glaucoma with "aplasia of the pectinate ligament", which does not respond to goniotomy. This idea is supported by BUSACCA and CARVALHO. (3) We find considerable variation in the gonioscopic appearance of these congenital glaucomas and think of them as different degrees of expression of the fetal condition of the angles and ordinarily try goniotomy in all of them of the infantile type.

There is further evidence that the decreased permeability of the Barkan membrane is a persistence of the fetal condition of the angle. KUPFER and ROSS have studied fetal eyes from 20 weeks to term. (5) They have compared the microscopic appearance with the facility of outflow. In fetuses under 7 months, there is a more or less continuous layer of endothelial cells covering the trabecular meshwork from the iris base to the corneal endothelium. In these eyes the average facility of outflow was 0.16. By the 8th gestational month, openings have appeared in this cellular covering and the average facility of outflow has increased to 0.24. The presence of this continuous cellular lining has been confirmed by the electron-microscopic studies of SMELSER and OZANICS and also by HANSSON and JERNDAL. (4, 14) Up to 8 months, they found a monolayer of endothelial cells that became discontinuous at term. It seems logical to think that the persistence of such a thin semipermeable layer of cells is responsible for infantile glaucoma.

A very superficial incision of this Barkan membrane results in a high percentage of cures of infantile glaucoma. This in itself is evidence of the membrane's impermeability. The height of the incision does not seem to be of critical importance. BARKAN, WORST, and we place our incisions anteriorly at the junction of the upper and middle third of the trabeculum. MAUMENEE, in the past, was making incisions through the posterior part of the membrane to cut the base of the iris and ciliary body free from the trabecular fibers. SCHEIE performed goniotomies without a contact lens so that the exact position of his incisions must have been quite variable. (10) Yet, statistically, the cure rate with these three methods was approximately the same. It therefore seems probable that a superficial incision at any point of the membrane will improve the facility of aqueous outflow. Obviously, the incision is safer if placed anteriorly under visual control.

Even a small goniotomy incision may be completely successful in normalizing pressure. Laboratory confirmation of this clinical observation comes from MAUMENEE and LANGHAM who obtained two eyes of an 8-month-old child 2h after death. Perfusion of the eyes revealed a facility of outflow of 0.10 in each. A 1-mm goniotomy was then performed with the tip of the perfusion needle. In each eye the facility of outflow promptly increased to 1.0.

Other typical findings in infantile glaucoma can be explained by the immature condition of all its tissues. Immature collagen can be stretched much more easily than mature collagen. This accounts for the enlargement of the infant globe under the influence of increased intraocular pressure. Descemet's membrane does not stretch as easily and eventually breaks, resulting in the sudden hazing of the cornea and the posterior corneal striae.

The decreasing effectiveness of goniotomy over the age of 1 year may be due to this maturing of the collagen cores of the meshwork. Certainly, the meshwork becomes thinner and less translucent with increasing age. It becomes more difficult to make a superficial cut in the trabecular meshwork without striking the underlying scleral sulcus. Deep incisions into the sclera have been shown to be less effective and intraocular hemorrhage is more common.

This same stretchability of immature collagen is responsible for another typical finding, the rapid cupping of the optic disk when pressure is elevated and the prompt decrease of that cupping when tensions have been normalized. Until the late 1960 s, it had been taught that disk-cupping was a late finding in congenital glaucoma. SUGAR stated in 1967, "Cupping of the optic disc does not occur early due to distensibility of the globe." (15) It is of considerable interest that BARKAN in 1948 described a case of congenital glaucoma whose pressure had been normalized by goniotomy. He stated, "It is interesting to note, incidentally, that the excavation of the nerve head almost disappeared following normalization of pressure. It appears that this effect is permanent." (2)

Using a smooth-domed Koeppe contact lens, SHAFFER and HETHERINGTON were able to see the optic nerve head despite severely hazed corneas. Not only was cupping of the optic disk an early sign of increased intraocular pressure, but regression of that cupping was so consistent with normalization of pressure that this has become a more important criterion for control than the height of the intraocular pressure. This phenomenon was first discussed in 1969 by SHAFFER and HETHERINGTON. (13) To account for these changes in cupping without damage to the neurons, it was suggested that the supporting tissue of the disk, the astroglial cells, might increase or decrease in number and also in volume and fluid content. When external pressure was applied to the eye during ophthalmoscopy, the cup size seemed to increase. This was never reported because the accompanying disk pallor prevented accurate observation. Now QUIGLEY has proved the matter experimentally. (8) He subjected fetal, neonatal, and adult eye bank eyes to perfusion pressure of 50 mm Hg over a 24-h period. The fetal and neonatal eyes showed obvious enlargement of the cups and bowing back of the lamina cribrosa. Mature eyes did not develop increase in cupping. Microscopic examination of these same optic nerves showed essentially no mature collagen in the fetal eyes and little at birth at the level of the lamina cribrosa. There was considerable mature collagen in the 12-year-old nerve and much more in the 49-year-old that he studied.

It is appropriate that this paper be closed as it started with a tribute to Otto BARKAN. His idea that the pathologic changes of infantile glaucoma are the result of an arrest in differentiation of the fetal eye seems to be true. The goniotomy technique devised by him is being used today without significant improvements. In these 40 years there have been many children rescued from darkness and living in the light because of his genius.

Reverences

(1) Barkan, O.: Operation for congenital glaucoma. Am. J. Ophthalmol. 25, 552 (1942)

(2) Barkan, O.: Goniotomy for the relief of congenital glaucoma. Br. J. Ophthalmol. 32, 701 (1948)

(3) Busacca, A.; Carvalho, C.: La gonioscopie du glaucome congenital. Ann Oculist. 201, 887 (1968)

(4) Hansson, H.; Jerndal, T.: Scanning electron microscopic studies on the development of the iridocorneal angle in human eyes. Invest Ophthalmol. 10, 252 (1971)

(5) Kupfer, C.; Ross, K.: The development of outflow facility in human eyes. Invest. Ophthalmol. 10(7), 513 (1971)

(6) Maumenee, A.: Further observations on the pathogenesis of congenital glaucoma. Trans. Am. Ophthalmol. Soc. 60, 140 (1962)

(7) Maumenee, A.: The pathogenesis of congenital glaucoma: A new theory. Trans. Am. Ophthalmol. 56, 507 (1958)

(8) Quigley, H.: The pathogenesis of reversible cupping in congenital glaucoma. Am. J. Ophthalmol. 84, 358 (1977)

(9) Sampaolesi, R.: Glaucoma. p. 411. Buenos Aires: Panamericana 1974

(10) Scheie, H.: Goniotomy in the treatment of congenital glaucoma. Arch. Ophthalmol. 42, 266 (1949)

(11) Seefelder, R.: Clinical and anatomical investigations of the pathology and therapy of congenital hydrophthalmos. Albrecht von Graefes Arch. Klin. Ophthalmol. 63, 205, 481 (1906)

(12) Shaffer, R.: Pathogenesis of congenital glaucoma. Trans. Am. Acad. Ophthalmol. Otolaryngol. 59, 297 (1955)

(13) Shaffer, R.; Hetherington, J.: The glaucomatous disk in infants. Am. J. Ophthalmol. 73, 929 (1969)

(14) Smelser, G.; Ozanics, V.: The development of the trabecular meshwork in primates. Am. J. Ophthalmol. 71, 366 (1971)

(15) Sugar, S.: The glaucomas. p. 285. New York: Hoeber-Harper 1957

(16) Worst, J.: The cause and treatment of congenital glaucoma. Trans. Am. Acad. Ophthalmol. Otolaryngol. 68, 766 (1964)

Carvalhs, Sampaolesi and Shaffei: Summary of Discussions on Congenital Glaucoma

Evaluation of Glaucoma Control

SAMPAOLESI and CARVALHO depend on applanation tonometry. SAMPAOLESI advises the use of Pentrane (METOXIFLUORANE) as the anesthetic agent. SHAFFER distrusts tonometry because of its marked variabilty in the anesthetized infant. He has found little difference between applanation and Schiotz readings. He and his group rely on ophthalmoscopy, believing that adequate pressure control usually results in a decrease in cupping. An increase in cupping always means inadequate control. SAMPAOLESI stressed that normal infant tensions average 10 mm Hg before the age of 12 months as he demonstrated in the Würzburg Symposium (1974). SAMPAOLESI, based on YTERBORG'S contribution, stresses the importance of applanation in children. Due to different scleral rigidity in children and adults, as was previously demonstrated, the intraocular pressure in children was equally low under local and general anesthesia. RAUTKE and COHAN (1976) confirmed SAMPAOLESI'S values for the intra ocular pressure in normal children under local and general anesthesia.

Trabeculotomy *vs* Goniotomy

Agreements: trabeculotomy and goniotomy give equivalently good results in congenital (infantile) glaucoma patients in the 1st year of life. In babies over the age of 12 months, trabeculotomy is considerably more effective than goniotomy and is also safer than goniotomy if corneal clouding prevents adequate visualization of the angles. CARVALHO and SAMPAOLESI tend to use trabeculotomy in all cases of congenital glaucoma.

Disagreements: SHAFFER believes goniotomy is a simpler, safer operation for use in infantile glaucoma leaving the eys relatively undisturbed for other procedures, if pressure again becomes elevated.

Classification of Congenital Glaucoma

In the classification of congenital glaucoma, problems arose in the terms used in describing the angles. SHAFFER restricts the term infantile glaucoma to eyes showing the gonioscopic and pathologic changes described in his paper. SAMPAOLESI and CARVALHO have a more elaborate classification of pathologic embryologic changes. These include eyes with marked mesodermal remnants that respond to goniotomy, which SHAFFER would classify as a mesodermal dysplasia like a partially expressed Axenfeld syndrome that does not respond well to goniotomy or trabeculotomy.

The areas of disagreement are partially semantic but may also result from different population groups. The South Americans see far more heavily pigmented eyes. Classification of these questions would be best accomplished by these observers examining the same patients. Then a logical attempt can be made to describe the pathology seen. A uniform classification is essential if we are to achieve a consensus on the preferred therapy for each condition.

FRANÇOIS: I agree with the observations of Dr. SHAFFER. In the majority of my cases of congenital glaucoma, I found a persistence of mesodermal meshwork and only in a minority of cases a high insertion of the iris. So, we can consider congenital glaucoma as an arrest in the development of the eye at the fetal age of more or less 7 months. And therefore I also agree with Dr. SAMPAOLESI, who found a high amount of reticulin and a low amount of collagen. Reticulin is, indeed, the precursor of collagen, and at the fetal age of 7 months one normally finds much more reticulin than collagen, which is another argument in favor of an arrest of development in congenital glaucoma. On the other hand, I never found an aplasia of the angle tissue.

When the cornea is sufficiently clear, I obtain the same results with goniotomy that others do with trabeculotomy, that is to say, nearly 80% of successful cases. In may experience, a goniotomy can be very well performed without a contact lens.

HETHERINGTON: To discuss pathology at this and future meetings, it is important to establish common terminology. Of value is a current study where structures are described by color, location, density, and contour as accurately as possible. The eyes are also photographed gonioscopically, and patients are given a comprehensive examination. Based on these findings, we hope to correlate trabeculectomy pathologic specimens. Surgical and medical therapy results will be related to clinical findings. Thus far, subtle variations in angle abnormalities have been seen in the congenital glaucoma group. In general, eyes with unusual anterior segment findings similar to Axenfeld syndrome, Riegers anomaly, and other obvious goniodysgenesic changes responded poorly to surgery of any kind. Sturge-Weber patients responded very poorly to surgical therapy. Goniotomy results were excellent (90% success) in infantile glaucoma eyes. A joint effort should be made to resolve the many unanswerec problems in this group of glaucomas.

In our experience, pressures in infants fluctuate without interference. Other factors associated with surgical preparation cause a greater degree of variation in pressure. For this reason, the optic nerve head changes are a more reliable sign of an uncontrolled situation. Cupping changes rapidly in the young.

LEYDHECKER: In my opinion, it would be dangerous to replace tonometry by disk observation, especially since the disk can change in appearance quite rapidly. We need all available parameters, i.e., tonometry, disk observation, the axial length of the globe measured by echography, and the observation of the parents, since recurrence of watering of the eye, increased light sensitivity, redness of the conjuctiva or haziness of the cornea can be well observed by the parents and would be indications for recurrence of hypertension. The task for the future will be to differentiate more accurately between the different types of congenital glaucoma and to find the appropriate surgical intervention for each condition.

KITAZAWA: Do you modify the goniotomy procedure depending on the appearance of the angle; in other words, do you place your incision in the same place regardless of the gonioscopic findings?

KOLKER: Our experience indicates the same results noted by Dr. SHAFFER, i.e., applanation and Schiotz readings under anesthesia are usually in very close agreement. The hand-held applanation tonometers, however, have a great advantage in that they can be frequently used in the awake infant, especially under 6 months of age.

HALBERG: Did you see cases where the eye looks externally like an eye with congenital glaucoma: large eye, large corneal diameter, but clear cornea and intraocular pressure under anesthesia by applanation? The membrane is visible in the angle by Koeppe gonioscopy, but the membrane is not continuous. I have seen an eye like this recently, the fellow eye was completely normal.
It seems that in all subscleral filtrating procedures it is essential to make an iridectomy that extends beyond the hole that we created. If the iridectomy is smaller than the hole, there is a change to clip the iris into the wound and to deform the pupil.

HARMS: I agree with Dr. SAMPAOLESI that Schlemm's canal is to be found in congenital glaucoma, but it is more difficult than in an adult glaucoma. There are three reasons.
1) The sclera is very thin
2) The sclera tissue is very plastic
3) There is no normal position of Schlemm's canal; the position can be on the ciliary body but also at greater distance in front of the ciliary body.

Careful preparation is necessary. If a repeated trabeculotomy or a trabeculectomy was not successful, I carried out a cyclodiathermy in some cases. Sometime I repeated this operation, in some cases with permanent decrease of the intraocular pressure.

KOLKER: I am concerned that the photographs shown by Dr. CARVALHO as cases poorly responsive to goniotomy appear to be the same ones that Dr. SHAFFER's photographs demonstrate are most responsive to goniotomy. (Our experience agrees with Dr. SHAFFER's that most cases of congenital primary infantile glaucoma appear responsive to goniotomy). The most frequent cases seen by Dr. CALVALHO seem to be the type Dr. SHAFFER (and we) seldom see.

ERNEST (to Dr. Sampaolesi): There are many variables affecting intraocular pressure in infants such as anesthetic agent, anesthesia level, Valsalva movement, etc. How are reliable pressures obtained?

ERNEST: If the infants with congenital glaucoma have trabecular membranes due to arrested development, then there must be another variable, that of aqueous secretion, accounting for the differences in extent and onset of the signs of the disease.

Earliest Visual Field Disturbances in Glaucoma

Stephen M. Drance

University of British Columbia, Department of Ophthalmology, 2550 Willow Street, Vancouver, B.C. V5Z 3N9, Canada

I have been asked to liaise between the Glaucoma Research Group of the International Perimetric Society, which has just debated the early field defects in glaucoma and their reversibility, and the International Glaucoma Club.

In the discussion of the earliest visual field disturbance in glaucoma, there were three reports describing a series of patients at risk who had normal visual fields and who developed glaucomatous visual field defects. Such patients obviously show the earliest perimetric changes. The concensus of the Glaucoma Research Group of the Internationl Perimetric Society appeared to be that the earliest defects are paracentral scotomata, which are relative to start with but can be present to a maximum luminosity from the onset. An entire nerve fiber bundle may be depressed so that the presence of a paracentral scotoma may manifest itself as a nasal step in the central portion of the visual field. There was also agreement that in a number of patients the peripheral and mid peripheral nasal steps can be the earliest manifestation of nerve fiber bundle damage. Temporal visual field defects and other sector-shaped defects may on occasion be the earliest signs of a glaucomatous defect. Combinations of the various early defects occur and more than one nerve fiber bundle may be affected from the beginning. Both central and peripheral nasal steps frequently have a localized scotoma that can be plotted above the nasal step, but at times the scotoma may not be plotted and the nasal step would therefore be the only manifestation of a nerve fiber bundle disturbance. The superior maximal luminosity disturbances tend to lie nearer fixation, whereas the inferior ones are further from fixation and a little more nasal in their distribution.

The paracentral scotomata are usually relative defects to start with, and such a relative disturbance may manifest itself as a localized increase in scatter or variation of responses or an actual relative wedge-shaped scotoma that is particularly significant when it assumes a nerve fiber bundle distribution. There was concensus that the earliest defects and also the later ones show fluctuation not necessarily related to the height of the intraocular pressure.

Attention was drawn to rotational movements of the eye that may account for the fluctuation or apparent disappearance of small relative and even absolute disturbances as a result of such rotational changes. One must therefore make sure that changes in such scotomata are not due to this perimetric artifact.

Studies of asymmetric patients whose fields in both eyes were considered normal showed that usually on the side of the larger cup and the higher intraocular pressure the isopters may be contracted and the blind spot somewhat enlarged when the two fields are compared. This may be a subtle perimetric change that has been suspected in the past and may have to be looked for again in the future.

In our own studies, 35 eyes of 30 patients developed definitive reproducible nerve fiber bundle defects when at least two visual field defects had previously been obtained without a central or peripheral defect being present. The scotomata had to be present on at least two successive occasions. Twenty-seven (77%) of the 35 eyes developed a paracentral scotoma when the visual field disturbance was first discovered. In nine (26 %) the paracentral scotoma was the only initial field defect present; eight of these were relative and one absolute. Twenty-six (75 %) of the 35 eyes showed a nasal step when the field was initially discovered to be defective, and in seven (20 %) of them the nasal step was the only initial defect and in two (6 %) the nasal step could only be found in the peripheral field. Of the 35 eyes, there were therefore nine (26 %) that showed only a paracentral defect and seven (20 %) that developed nasal steps central or peripheral as the only initial field defect. The remaining 19 (54 %) had a combination of paracentral defects with a nasal step or a sector defect when the visual field first developed. It is of interest that the temporal sector-shaped defect, although accompanied by a nasal step, was in fact present at the very first abnormal visual field examination and may therefore be the only visual field disturbance present.

From the perimetric point of view, it would seem desirable to screen with a stimulus that is slightly supraliminal for the area to be tested. The entire central field should be screened with emphasis (kinetically or statically) on the nasal portion of the central, mid peripheral, and peripheral areas. Such screening should also include a plot of the peripheral isopter so as to find the uncharacteristic first field defects.

There was concensus that to screen the visual field the screening techniques and the equipment must make it possible for all areas of risk to be screened. Once a defective area is suggested by the screening, all subsequent defects have to be located and fully quantitated in terms of their position, shape, size, and depth. This requires quite a different technique from screening and requires time and good perimetry. It was the feeling that screening might shortly become automated, but the quantitative perimetry necessary for the management of the glaucoma patient is unlikely to be automated reliably in the immediate future.

A statistical analysis of the nasal portion of the visual field was presented by Professor Zingirian and our own group. Both studies showed that small nasal steps can occur in normals who are usually less than 4° in extent and lack reproducibility.

It was demonstrated that the earliest perimetric defects, which are predominantly expressions of nerve fiber bundle defects, may not be the earliest psychovisual disturbances in glaucoma. Color vision was shown to be disturbed in the yellow-blue and green-blue functions. Such disturbances could be related in severity with the severity of the visual field disturbances, even when the visual acuity remained normal. The color vision work showed that patients with elevated pressures without field defects had poorer color vision performance than normals of the same age and sex. Those who subsequently developed a visual field defect belonged to the worst group of color vision disturbances among the ocular hypertensives so that the possibility of using color parameters for predicting subsequent field loss was a possibility. The receptive field-like functions were also shown to be disturbed in glaucoma patients and sometimes preceded the appearance of nerve fiber loss. These studies pointed out that whereas nerve fiber bundle loss undoubtedly occurred in glaucoma, it should not confine our thinking and prevent us from looking at other sensory disturbances that may be disturbed earlier, predict nerve fiber bundle disturbance, and may show loss of function at a stage that is yet reversible. Measurements utilizing pupilography and the use of grating patterns might also be helpful in this regard.

The other main topic of discussion dealt with reversibility of glaucomatous visual field defects. Difficulties and pitfalls of studying reversibility were very clearly outlined, among them the spontaneous variability of the visual field defect, the rotational movement of the eye, the refractive changes of the eye, and the multiple etiology of nerve fiber bundle defects where someone had to be certain that the reversibility was a phenomenon over and above the normal variability of the visual field. Variability seems to be greater in areas that have already been partially damaged. It seemed to be the concensus that a small proportion of field defects did show reversibility, and it was more likely to occur in the young and those who do not show retinal nerve fiber loss or advanced disk changes and was also likely to occur in those who had high intraocular pressures that were considerably lowered. Reversibility could also be observed without any pressure reduction. Our Japanese colleagues demonstrated the use of equipment that allowed the plotting of visual fields by direct viewing of the fundus, usually done on a fundus camera. These techniques open new horizons for perimetry, not only of the glaucomas but many other disease states.

Attention was also drawn to the fact that there were many causes other than glaucoma for nerve fiber bundle disturbances and that patients who have glaucoma are quite likely to develop other disease processes that should always be looked for and remembered, particularly when a discrepancy in the appearance of the visual field and that of the optic nerve was present.

There was general concensus that the appearance of the disk and the plotting of the visual field should not be in any way mutually exclusive. Both have an important part to play in the recognition of the glaucomas at their earliest stages.

Kinetic Perimetry: Interobserver Variations

Nassim Calixto, Yehuda Waisberg, Geralda P. Costa, Maria A. Gomes

1177, Grão Mogol, Belo Horizonte, Brasil

Introduction

Our purpose in this paper is the study of visual field variations in the same eye by two different examiners. Perimetry is a subjective examination and therefore exposed to wide variations dependent not only on the patient but also on the previous knowledge of the examiner of the several visual field changes, fortuitously present, and on his ability to pick them up.

Goldmann in different papers has emphasized that "good perimetry, particularly kinetic perimetry is an art which is not very common." In the study of glaucoma, perimetry is in clear-cut contrast to tonometry and ophthalmoscopy 'also exposed to variations between observers' which are objective methods and independent from subjective co-operation of the patient for their attainment. The subjective factors should be kept in mind in the interpretation and judgment of the possible and frequent changes of visual fields obtained from more than one observer.

Material and Methods

Fifty-four glaucomatous patients (104 eyes; 34 women and 20 men ranging in age from 10 to 65, with and without visual field defects) were studied by two technicians with long experience in kinetic perimetry; the instrument used was the Goldmann Perimeter 940 (Haag-Streit); both technicians followed, step by step, the same routine in the examinations as well as the rules contained in the instruction manual of the perimeter.

Special Care

1) Refraction of each eye made by one of us (N.C.) with the best near vision correction for 30 cm (perimeter's radius); as far as possible, the spheric equivalent was used instead of spheric-cylindric combinations.

2) The miotics were stopped 24 - 48 h before each examination to keep the horizontal pupil diameter ⩾ 2.50 mm; additional phenylephrine drops (10%) were used to dilate when necessary.
3) Diamox (250 - 750 mg/day) was used to maintain the intraocular pressure (IOP) below 25 mm Hg (applanation) when necessary.
4) In general, the right eye was examined before the left.
5) The targets used were: size 1 (0.25 mm^2) unchanged; intensity decreasing from 4e to 1e.
6) In general 24 h interval were kept between the two examinations; however, ten patients (20 eyes) were examined on the same day (first examination in the morning and the second in the afternoon).
7) Technician G. made the first examination in 34 patients (65 eyes) and technician M. made the first examination in 20 patients (39 eyes). The first technician, after her examination, prepared the graph for the second examiner, registering the targets used in the first examination, but the second technician did not see the results obtained in the first examination.
8) In each graph of visual field, the technicians mentioned their "impressions" about the quality of information obtained from each patient (each eye) during the examination: in 12 cases of the total sample (104), the "impressions" were in disagreement (11%).

Pupil Diameter

The mean pupillary diameters obtained in the first and second examinations, in both eyes, are presented in Table 1.

Table 1. Pupillary diameter

1 st examination	2nd examination	Paired *t*	*P*
OD 3.67 ± 0.86	3.75 ± 1.06	-0.71	-
OS 3.74 ± 0.92	3.65 ± 1.11	0.63	-

OD, oculus dexter; OS, oculus sinister

The differences between the pupillary diameters in the two examinations were not significant; this finding is important to exclude as a frequent cause of error in the evaluation of the visual fields.

Visual Fields Classification

Initially, we analyzed the total sample (pool) and then divided the visual fields into four groups according to the following classification:

Normal visual fields 55 eyes (53%)
Abnormal visual fields
Type I 26 eyes (25%)
Type II 09 eyes (09%)
Type III 14 eyes (13%)

The visual fields obtained by the two technicians on the same day (10 patients = 20 eyes) were also studied separately to check the differences or similarities in relation to those performed with the time interval of 24 h. Unfortunately, we had to stop the double examination on the same day due to the frequent feeling of visual fatigue mentioned by some patients.

Evaluation of the Visual Fields

We had great difficulties in establishing the criteria for comparison of the visual fields. We adopted a quantitative and a clinical method for checking the visual field differences.

1) To analyze quantitatively the variations between the two observers, we calculated the areas of each isopter and of the blind spot in all the graphs. The areas were determined with the Compensating Planimeter KP-25 (Koizumi). The areas were measured at least two times for each isopter, and the arithmetic means were used for analysis.
2) The clinical criterion consisted of putting the different graphs made by the two technicians for the same eye side by side and judging the clinical differences. The results were:
   a) Similar visual fields 87 eyes (83.5%)
   b) Small differences in visual fields 12 eyes (11.5%)
   c) Large differences in visual fields 5 eyes (5.0%)

Results and Comments

The statistical analysis of the total planimetric data (R.E. and L.E. separately) showed significant differences for all the isopters and also for the blind spot, for both right and left eyes (Table 2). The values obtained by technician G. were always greater than those obtained by technician M. for all isopters. The opposite occurred in relation to the blind spot in both eyes. This finding was systematically present in all the groups analyzed (Tables 3 and 4). This fact suggests a systematic difference between the two observers in the examination technique or in the registration of the correspondent points to the stimuli perceptions on the graph.

Table 2. Total sample

		No. of eyes	Technician G. Mean ± 1 SD	Technician M. Mean ± 1 SD	t	P<
4/1	OD	52	1166.8 ± 316.0	1103.0 ± 369.0	2.34	0.01
	OS	52	1161.0 ± 334.0	1094.0 ± 391.0	2.66	0.01
3/1	OD	51	634.0 ± 231.0	563.0 ± 253.0	3.80	0.001
	OS	52	630.0 ± 255.0	576.0 ± 272.0	3.28	0.002
2/1	OD	52	251.0 ± 149.0	214.0 ± 121.0	3.55	0.001
	OS	52	254.0 ± 164.0	228.0 ± 154.0	2.22	0.02
1/1	OD	32	74.0 ± 57.0	61.0 ± 38.0	1.94	0.05
	OS	30	81.0 ± 57.0	68.0 ± 46.5	1.75	0.05
Blind spot	OD	46	16.0 ± 5.7	19.0 ± 9.8	-3.69	0.001
	OS	47	16.0 ± 7.8	19.4 ± 6.4	-4.04	0.001

OD, oculus dexter; OS, oculus sinister.

As we know for the determination of the isopters, the target comes from a blind to a seeing area (from outside to inside); for the blind spot the target comes from inside to outside according to the same principle. The observed difference was, therefore probably due to the different reaction time and/or different speed in the movement of the targets between the two technicians.

Table 3. Different groups according to the visual vield changes

	Normal					Group I				
	No. of eyes	Tech. G. Mean ± 1 SD	Tech. M. Mean ± 1 SD	t	P<	No. of eyes	Tech. G. Mean ± 1 SD	Tech. M. Mean ± 1 SD	t	P<
4/1	55	1351.0 ± 145.0	1356.0 ± 243.0	0.21	-	26	1126.0 ± 214.0	971.0 ± 212.0	4.51	0.001
3/1	54	789.0 ± 154.0	741.0 ± 196.5	2.69	0.005	26	494.0 ± 154.0	423.0 ± 146.0	2.50	0.01
2/1	55	347.0 ± 128.0	306.0 ± 97.0	3.58	0.001	24	143.0 ± 104.0	125.0 ± 94.0	1.83	0.05
1/1	51	85.0 ± 59.0	76.0 ± 47.0	1.83	0.05	8	49.0 ± 30.0	32.0 ± 14.0	1.79	-
Blind spot	55	15.0 ± 2.8	18.0 ± 4.0	-5.66	0.001	26	15.7 ± 3.5	18.0 ± 4.4	-2.62	0.01

Visual Field Groups

The results of the analysis of the groups of normal and pathologic visual fields are presented separately in Table 3. In general, the same systematic difference between the two technicians persisted for both isopters and the blind spot. However, small statistical differences appeared: in the normal group and in group III the isopter 4/1 showed no significant difference between the two technicians; the same happened for the isopter 1/1 in group I and for the blind spot in group II.

Visual Fields in the Same Day (Table 4)

During the investigation, ten patients (20 eyes) had a double perimetry (morning and afternoon) on the same day by the two technicians. Technicians G. and M. both examined five patients each in the morning (first examination). The statistical analysis showed no significant differences in the examined parameters (with one exception for the isopter 2/1). Nevertheless, the systematic differences between the two technicians, as discussed before, were also noted.

We had planned to increase the number of cases of double perimetry on the same day, but we stopped this procedure on the belief that the visual fatigue reported by some patients after the second perimetry might sensitively change the results or

Table 3. (Continued)

	Group II					Group III				
		Tech. G.	Tech. M.				Tech. G.	Tech. M.		
	No. of eyes	Mean ± 1 SD	Mean ± 1 SD	t	P <	No. of eyes	Mean ± 1 SD	Mean ± 1 SD	t	P <
4/1	11	1083.0 ± 208.0	861.0 ± 201.0	7.34	0.001	14	562.0 ± 305.0	514.0 ± 241.0	1.11	-
3/1	11	528.0 ± 176.0	404.0 ± 138.0	3.90	0.002	12	261.0 ± 170.0	243.0 ± 154.0	6.30	0.001
2/1	11	175.0 ± 103.0	129.0 ± 106.0	2.31	0.02	11	76.0 ± 67.0	84.0 ± 97.0	-4.39	0.002
1/1	-	-	-	-	-	-	-	-	-	-
Blind spot	9	24.0 ± 1.9	29.0 ± 2.2	-1.20	-	-	-	-	-	-

introduce additional variation. However, the statistical analysis showed exactly the opposite: in this small sample, in contrast to the major one studied with a 24 h interval, the differences were statistically insignificant. In this group, 4 out of 20 eyes showed clinical differences between the two observers, while 13 of 84 eyes showed clinical differences in the visual field examinations performed with a 24 h interval. The difference was not significant ($\chi^2 = 0.29$).

Table 4. Visual fields performed on the same day

	No. of eyes	Tech. G. Mean ± 1 SD	Tech. M. Mean ± 1 SD	t	P <
4/1	20	1208.9 ± 335.6	1149.6 ± 311.8	1.34	-
3/1	20	629.9 ± 278.3	592.2 ± 245.1	1.30	-
2/1	19	256.4 ± 171.0	219.3 ± 134.5	1.77	0.05
1/1	10	75.3 ± 51.8	69.1 ± 38.1	0.51	-
Blind spot	17	20.3 ± 14.1	24.2 ± 17.0	-1.73	-

Conclusions

We think that the main conclusions of this work are:

1) An individual coefficient of variation is always present in the search of the visual fields even with an expert technician.
2) This fact was responsible for the statistically significant differences found in the comparison of the examinations of the isopteric areas and of the blind spot areas of the visual fields performed by the two technicians in each eye.
3) However, the clinical significance of this difference is generally small when the conditions of the examination are kept constant.
4) In only five eyes (5%) of our sample were large differences between the two observers found on clinical grounds.

References

Berry et al.-: An evaluation of differences between two observers plotting and measuring visual fields. Can. J. Ophthalmol. 1, 297 (1966).

Automatic Perimetry in Secondary Prevention of Glaucoma

Bo Bengtsson and C.E.T. Krakau

University Eye Clinic, Department of exp. Ophthalmology, S- 22185 Lund, Sweden

During the last few years, an automatic perimeter has been developed and tested at the Department of Experimental Ophthalmology in Lund (3, 4). A great deal of clinical experience was gained, and a trial of the logic for glaucoma visual field screening (2) in a population survey was considered appropriate.

Material

All persons born from 1907 up to and including 1921 and resident in the district served by the Dalby Community Care Center were listed in December 1976. The list was arranged according to the residential addresses and kept up to date by means of weekly reports from the County Council on departures from the district and deaths. Following this directory, the inhabitants were contacted and offered repeated ophthalmologic examinations. Attempts at persuasion were avoided and only persons able and willing to attend within a few weeks were included in the survey. Seven patients known to be undergoing antiglaucomatous therapy were not invited. There were no demonstrable field defects in this group.

Of 733 persons invited, 572 (78%) took part in the survey. The rate of attendance was largely independent of age and sex. Automatic perimetry was attempted in 1135 eyes (567 right and 568 left). The field screening was completed in 1121 eyes (561 right and 560 left) of 568 individuals. Fourteen screenings were not completed because of nystagmus, unsatisfactory co-operation, or for trivial reasons.

Methods

Sphygmomanometric measurements of systemic blood pressure, determination of visual acuity, subjective refraction, automatic perimetry, fundus photography, indirect ophthalmoscopy, slit-lamp examination, and Goldmann tonometry were attempted in every case. Perimetric data handling was entirely automatic, and other data were immediately recorded on special forms. Transfer to magnetic tape and further processing were performed at the computer center in Lund. Perimetry and photography were conducted by two alternating assistants - ophthalmoscopy, slit-lamp examination, and tonometry by one of the authors (BB).

Perimeter

The perimeter described by HEIJL and KRAKAU (3) was used. Sixty-four test points are fixed in a pattern of concentric circles at 5°, 10°, and 15° eccentricity. At 20° there are only eight points, placed as shown in Fig. 1. At each test point there is a LED (light-emitting diode) that can be ordered to emit light at 16 levels. The relation of luminance between two consecutive levels is 1:2. One further light spot is used for fixation control. This is projected onto the perimeter screen, adjusted to fall in the blind spot area, and lit at random intervals at an average of 1/9 of all trials. If the patient keeps his fixation it cannot be seen. The patient signals that he has perceived a light by pressing a button.

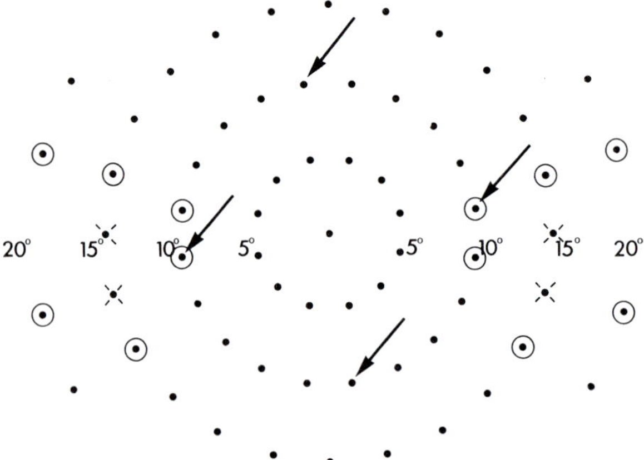

Fig. 1. Location of test points. The threshold is first determined at the four places indicated by arrows. When one or two of the points (⋇) and, eventually, one or two of the points (⊙) are not seen, the blind spot is denoted normal. (The right group refers to the right eye, and vice versa).

Test Logic

The test procedure is similar to the programs for glaucoma screening by manual perimetry as used by ARMALY, DRANCE, and others. However, the points tests are chosen in random order in the computerized version. [Minor changes only have been made in the program as used by HEIJL (2)]. The threshold is at first determined at four points on the 10° circle (Fig. 1). If, at a certain point, a target is seen, it is shown the next time on a one-step fainter level and vice versa. The target perceived is accepted as the threshold when the process has changed its direction three times.

A supraliminal test value is calculated from the thresholds of the first four points and used as starting level for the remaining test points. If, at any point, this level is seen, this point is not tested again; if not, the test level is increased by one step. If this level is seen, this point is not tested again; if not seen, the process starts from the very highest intensity level and passes, step by step, to lower intensities and ends as soon as the light is no longer seen (Fig.2).

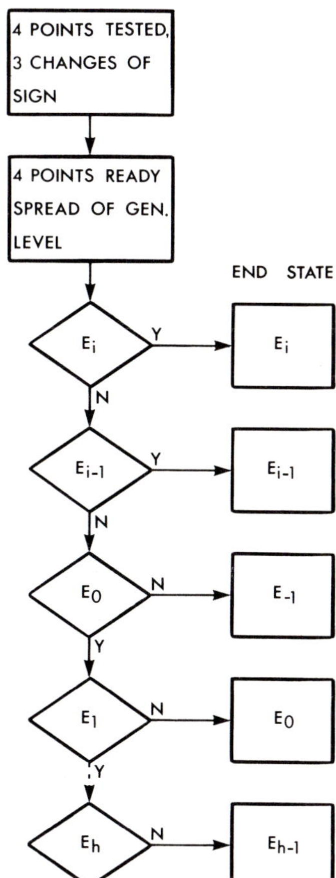

Fig.2. Flow diagram showing the course of testing one point. E_i, starting level; E_0, highest intensity level; Y, seen; N, not seen.

Conditions

As a rule the blind spot stimuli for fixation control were directed toward a point about 2cm temporal and inferior to the test diode 15° temporal to the fixation light. An individual adjustment was resorted to only when an anomalous position of the blind spot was suspected. Only spheric glasses were used to correct for near vision and no special measures were taken to secure dark adaptation. The instructions to the subjects (to fixate the red light and to press the button whenever a white light is seen) were kept as few and simple as possible. The assistant remained in the room for a while but left its as soon as she felt assured that co-operation was satisfactory.

Presentation of Results

The results were presented by means of a "keyboard-printer" (Silent 700, Texas Instruments). The printout of one field chart required less than 1 min. The type of representation was similar to that described by Krakau (5).

Interpretation

A test point was considered seen if it had ended on a level not more than one step lower than the initial one. Up to four points not seen in the blind spot area (Fig. 1) were accepted as a normal blind spot. If the blind spot was missed and, in addition, the blind spot check light seen more than five times, the test was regarded as unreliable.

A reliable test was considered normal if all points outside the normal blind spot were seen (otherwise abnormal). If a reliable test was normal the eye was classed as negative.

When a reliable, abnormal test was obtained in an eye with a known field defect or with a defect that could be attributed to an ophthalmoscopic finding, the eye was considered positive and not further investigated. With this exception, all unreliable or abnormal tests were repeated, as shown in the flow diagram (Fig. 3).

If the first reliable test was abnormal, a proposed defect was assumed. If such a defect was followed by a similar one in the same eye, the points outside the normal blind spot were compared. If at least one of those points was "not seen" in both tests, the second test had a confirmed defect, and the screening was considered positive. If a proposed defect was not reproduced at any point in the second test, the screening was considered negative. The classification of an eye as "positive" or "negative" followed rules so strict that the computer was entrusted with it. The operatur made the decision of a retest, but even this task could have been left to the computer.

Results

The background illumination was in three cases $0.1\,cd/m^2$, in all others $1\,cd/m^2$. There was no difference in the level reached between the first (right) and the second (left) eye. Thus, there was no indication of an insufficient adaptation. The time needed for a test session (one eye) was less than 3 min in 90% of all normal eyes. The field screening was completed in 1121 eyes. The screening was considered negative in 1079 eyes and positive in 42 eyes (4%).

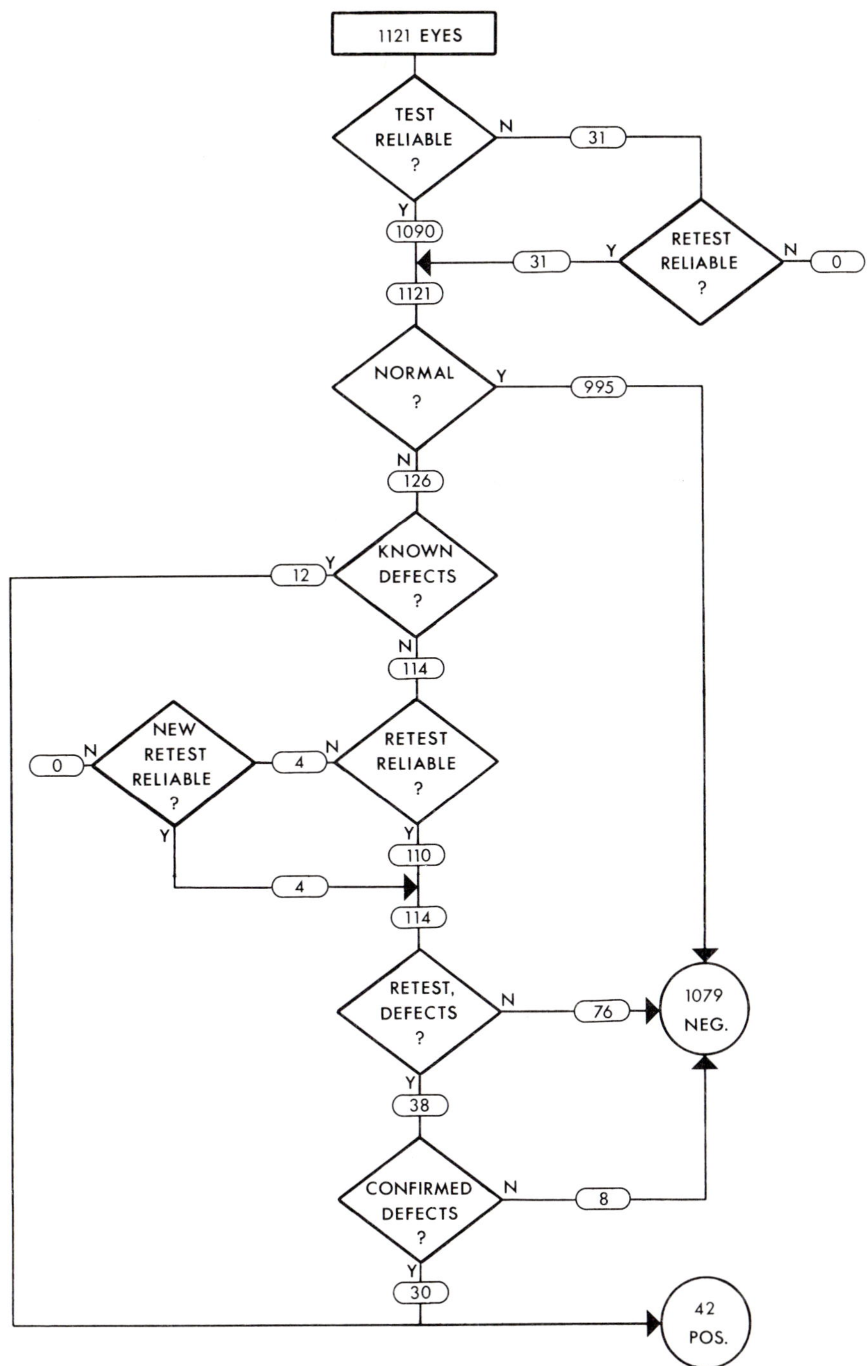

Fig.3. Flow diagram, followed when classifying a tested eye as positive or negative. The number of eyes subjected to test, retest, etc. is encircled.

Three known field defects were all spotted by the automatic perimeter. We also soon learned to expect relative temporal defects or enlarged blind spots in highly myopic eyes with posterior staphyloma and/or peripapillary atrophy. In seven such cases (nine eyes), the screening was terminated when the initial test had shown a proposed defect.

The field screening was considered to be a false positive in five cases (seven eyes). One subject could not be prevented from "over fixating." One deaf person was an excellent lip reader and therefore left by mistake without adequate instructions in the dark room. In three cases, external causes partly blocking the sight in one eye were overlooked and therefore not eliminated.

From our point of view, the actual yield of the survey was 23 unknown and unexpected defects '13 glaucomatous and ten others' described in Table 1. They were reproducible and also possible to verify by Goldmann perimetry, if not by ophthalmoscopy. Their extension was in general adequately mapped by the "automatic" field chart.

Table 1. Unknown and unexpected visual field defects

	Cases	Eyes
Glaucomatous scotomata		
Arcuate in both eyes	1	2
Arcuate in one eye and circumscribed in the other	1	2
Circumscribed in both eyes	1	2
Arcuate in one eye	2	2
Circumscribed in one eye	5	5
Other scotomata		
Homonymous paracentral	2	4
Circumscribed paracentral, of unknown etiology	1	1
Circumscribed paracentral, corresponding with small but obvious fundus lesion	5	5

The 13 glaucomatous defects were found in eyes with pathologic excavation of the disk and/or small hemorrhages on its margin 'except in one case in which the pressure was high (and the defect on the increase).

The blind spot was "missed" in 11% of all reliable tests. This rate was 9% even if the fixation was good (i.e., the check light seen $\leqslant$ 2 times) and still less than 40% when the fixation check light was seen exactly five times. Little would therefore have been gained by considering tests unreliable (and in need of repetition) more often than was actually done.

Discussion

When first recognizable, glaucomatous field defects are small, circumscribed, deep scotomas, which may appear anywhere in the central field (1). The perimeter is unable to separate absolute scotomas from deep relative ones, and the blind spot area is treated in exactly the same way as the rest of the paracentral field. Any attempt to detect defects smaller than the blind spot must obviously be futile since perimetry cannot be performed incessantly. The fact that the probability of detecting the blind spot by automatic perimetry is as high as about 0.9 should therefore mean that the method amply fulfills any reasonable demands on sensitivity. Surely the detection of 23 small and unexpected defects does not contradict this conclusion. The rate of verified defects not warranting ophthalmologic care was greater than might be desired but, of course, a natural and inevitable consequence of the high sensitivity. Our main concern was, however, specificity, since a high rate of false positives might easily become a major obstacle. We were therefore much relieved to find that after retesting very few, if any, unexplained false positives remained. We conclude that the procedure of automatic perimetry in the form applied is quick, sensitive, specific, and dependable.

Summary

Automatic perimetry was performed in 1121 eyes of 568 subjects born from 1907 up to and including 1921 and resident in a certain small area. Unreliable or abnormal tests were repeated. The average number of tests per person was 2.25. About 90% of all tests were done in less than 3 min. The screening was considered negative in 1079 eyes and positive in 42 eyes (4%). Thirteen of these were glaucomatous defects. There were few, if any, unexplained false positives. We concluded that the method is quick, sensitive, specific, and dependable. The apparatus is simple to manage and inexpensive to run.

References

(1) Aulhorn, E.; Harms, H.: Early visual field defects in glaucoma. In: Glaucoma-Symposium, Tutzing Castle 1966. pp 151-186. Basel, New York: Karger 1967

(2) Heijl, A.: Automatic perimetry in glaucoma visual field screening. A clinical study. Albrecht von Graefes Arch. Klin. Ophthalmol. 200, 21-37 (1976)

(3) Heijl, A.; Krakau, C.E.T.: An automatic static perimeter, design and pilot study. Acta Ophthalmol. (Kbh.) 53, 293-310 (1975)

(4) Heijl, A.; Krakau, C.E.T.: An automatic perimeter for glaucoma visual field screening and control. Construction and clinical cases. Albrecht von Graefes Arch. Klin. Ophthalmol. 197, 13-23 (1975)

(5) Krakau, C.E.T.: Aspects on the design of an automatic perimeter. Acta Ophthalmol. (Kbh.) (in press) (1978)

Pros and Cons of Quick-Tests in Glaucoma Perimetry

Elfriede Aulhorn

University Eye Hospital, Schleichstraße 12, D-7400 Tübingen, Germany (FRG)

The perimetric examination in glaucoma must perform three different tasks:

1) The most complete detection possible of early defects, including defects of slight extent as well as those in unexpected locations in the visual field. This examination must be at least so thorough that, in cases where no scotoma is found, the examiner can feel justified in saying that he is dealing with a normal visual field.
2) A follow-up of these defects, which must lead to the ascertainment of whether or not the defects increase. This is of decisive importance concerning the question as to the effectiveness or necessity of therapeutic measures.
3) An exact topographic registration of advanced glaucomatous visual field defects, so that possible deteriorations can also be determined here.

Whereas an examination within a central visual field area is sufficient for the first and second tasks, an examination of the whole visual field is necessary for the third. The central visual field area should have a range of at least 20° on all sides, since all kinds of early defects are to be found in this central visual field sector, whether they are small, spot-like Bjerrum's scotomas or early forms of the nasal step.

All three perimetric tasks can be performed manually or automatically. The advantages of the automatic examination are as follows:

It saves time for the doctor who does not have to sit performing the examination himself. This is not true as far as the patient is concerned; on the contrary, it tires him just as much or even more so because he must answer questions for the computer.

It eliminates the influence of different examiners but is not better than a very good examiner.

It offers the test point in random order.

It is much more suitable for the registration and storage of the results.

As with manual perimetry, automatic perimetry can also reach any degree of accuracy through increasing the number of examination points. The investigation of more points is more time-consuming for the patient in automatic as well as in manual perimetry.

Consequently, I believe that the problem that should be discussed is not the question of whether to perform an automatic or non-automatic examination, but rather concerning the following aspects:

1) First a quick test followed by a detailed examination
2) A quick test only
3) A detailed examination only.

All three methods may or may not be performed automatically.

A quick test using a simple instrument specially made for this test has the great advantage that it can be carried out as often as necessary. Detailed perimetry will only be done rarely in private practice since it either requires a large and expensive automatic perimeter or a good hemisphere perimeter operated by a very well-trained examiner familiar with the problems of glaucomatous visual field defects.

In my opinion, the task of detecting early glaucomatous defects can certainly be accomplished by a quick test instrument. We should now discuss how the glaucoma quick test should be designed to detect a maximum of early defects. To do this, it is first of all important to know what kind of early defects there are, in which ways they can change, and how they differ from defects in advanced stages.

In classifying the degree of severity of the glaucomatous defects, five stages of development result of their own accord, whereby the first stage corresponds to the beginning of visual field damage in the form of relative defects, and the fifth stage is equivalent to the final condition (Fig.1). In most cases, the functional disturbance can only be determined with certainty in the second stage, in the form of often very small visual field defects, frequently lying close to the center. Such scotomas in the second stage are usually absolute and irreversible already, and once they have been found and their location in the visual field is consequently known, they are perimetrically well-reproducible.

Whether or not every early glaucomatous spot-like defect has been preceded by a relative defect, as characterized in stage one, is not known for certain. It would also appear that there are remissions in stage 1. This is, however, difficult to prove, since relative defects are fundamentally more difficult to determine perimetrically than absolute defects. In this way, a change in diameter of the pupil or in the correction used in perimetry can influence the height of profile courves, just as a variation in attention may do so. In the resulting individual scatter, areas of sensorially reduced light difference sensitivity can easily remain unrecognized.

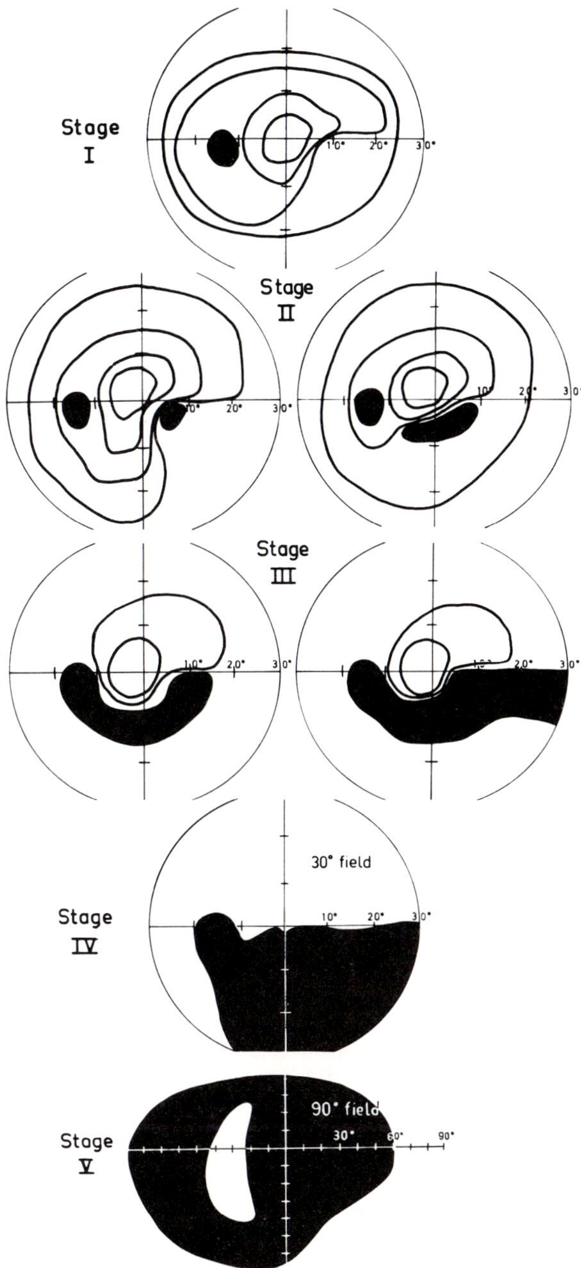

Fig.1. The five stages of development of glaucomatous field defects using the example of a defect beginning in the lower half of the visual field. In stages II and III, two possible defects are shown for each stage.

In our experience, the spot-like defects of the second stage very often lie in an area with normal function. In profile perimetry, these then appear as steeply sloping, deep indentations in the profile curve (Fig.2). They can expand more or less quickly and take on arcuate shape, frequently without relative defects being found previously in the newly damaged areas. This could be an indication that the first spot-like defects can also appear without preceding relative damage.

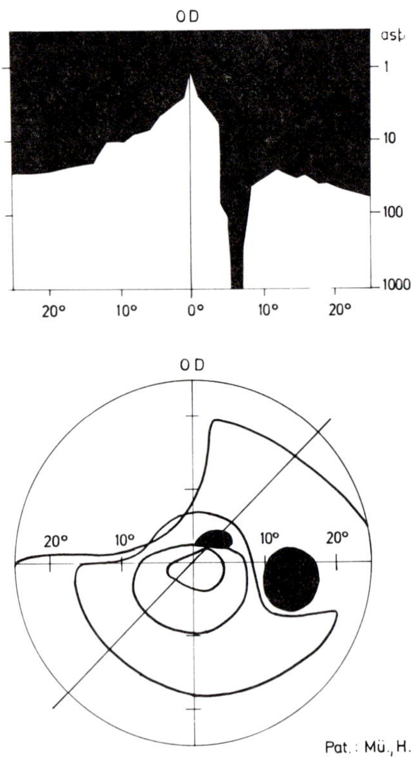

Fig.2. Typical early glaucomatous field defect; there is an absolute scotoma with normal retinal sensitivity in the immediate vicinity.

However, this may be the first perimetric sign of functional disturbance that can be determined with certainty, is the small, spot-like defect of the second stage. The perimetric method, therefore, that can determine such scotomas most quickly and with the greatest certainty, seems to me to be the best method. A problem for every screening method is the uncertainty of location and the often very slight extent of the scotoma. The frequency distribution of scotoma location in glaucoma can be seen in Fig.3, which shows the results of 400 visual fields, with spot-like scotomas. The visual field record form, used for the registration of all 400 visual fields, was divided into small fields, and with every scotoma the fields touched were marked. We can see that the majority of scotomas lying superior appear closer to the center, and those lying inferior further from it and predominantly nasal in the visual field. If the scotoma location is related to the underlying nerve fiber damage in the region of the optic disk, then it can be assumed that this, too, is either superior or inferior at different positions (Fig.4).

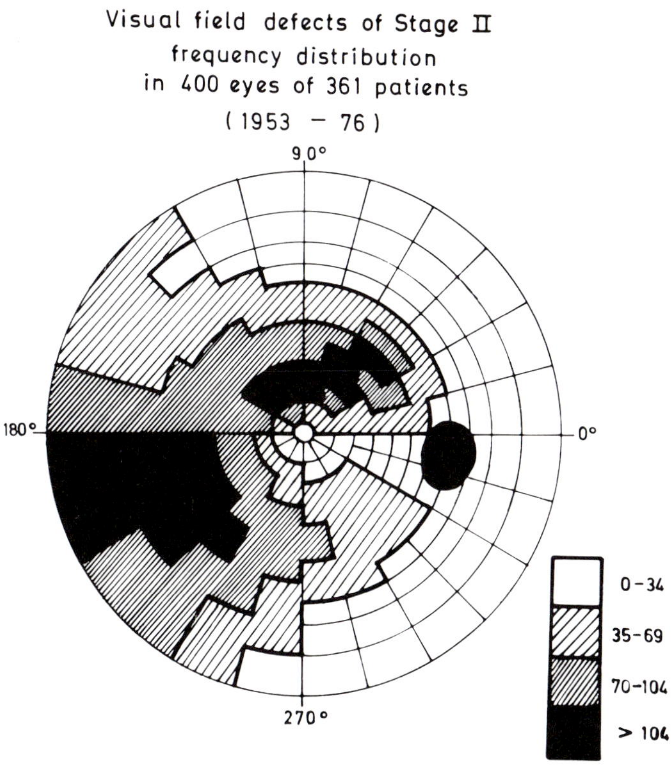

Fig.3. Visual field defect of stage II. Frequency distribution of the location of the scotomas, found in 400 eyes of 361 patients.

The defects are often very small, about the size of the blind spot or considerably smaller. A good method of glaucoma perimetry must, therefore, in the crucial visual field area have examination points lying as close together as possible. The closer they lie, the greater the probability is of discovering the small defects as well. On the other hand, however, the examination lasts all the longer, the greater the number of examination points. The longer it lasts, the more likely it is that the patient will be overtaxed, and consequently the doctor decides just as rarely to do a perimetric examination.

The best solution for both patient and doctor is probably the so-called quick test, which is suitable for sifting out all suspicious cases, so that these can then be submitted to a thorough perimetric examination. With a combined method of examination such as this, the big sacrifice of time involved in a thorough examination would subsequently only be necessary for those cases with actual pathologic visual fields.

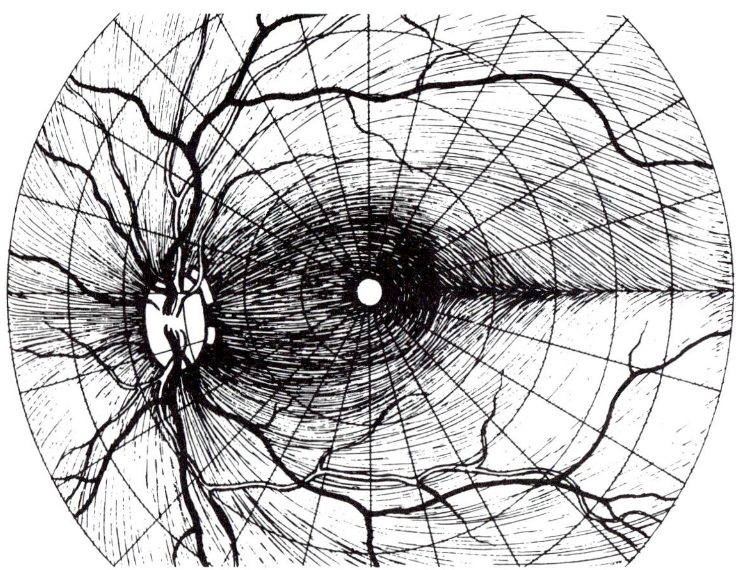

Fig.4. Nerve fiber pathway in the retina according to Harrington. At the temporal edge of the disk, the nerve fiber bundles are marked where, according to the frequency distribution of glaucomatous field defects, the first damage is expected to be.

The early defects of stage two are now accessible to a shortened form of perimetry in the form of a quick test, because 'as discussed' they are absolute defects from a very early stage. It is, therefore, in my opinion justified to perform the quick test with only one or rather two test point luminances, which should, however, be fairly high above threshold. I would recommend a luminance of 100 asb (or 32 cd/m^2) and 10 asb (or 3.2 cd/m^2) for this purpose. The time saved by omitting change in luminance should then, however, be used to benefit the number of examination points, to increase the likelihood of discovering all scotomas with a close net of points.

At how many and at which points in the visual field should the technical designer offer the test points of a quick test? The problem is indicated in Fig.5, which shows that the quick test can only give reliable results if it uses a somewhat overly fine mesh for the division into healthy and pathologic visual fields (Fig.5e), for on no account should diseased visual fields slip through the sieve, i.e., into the group of healthy fields (Fig.5c). It is, however, just as undesirable that, apart form the pathologic fields, too many healthy ones remain in the sieve, i.e., appear in the group of diseased visual fields (Fig.5d), since then an unnecessarily high number

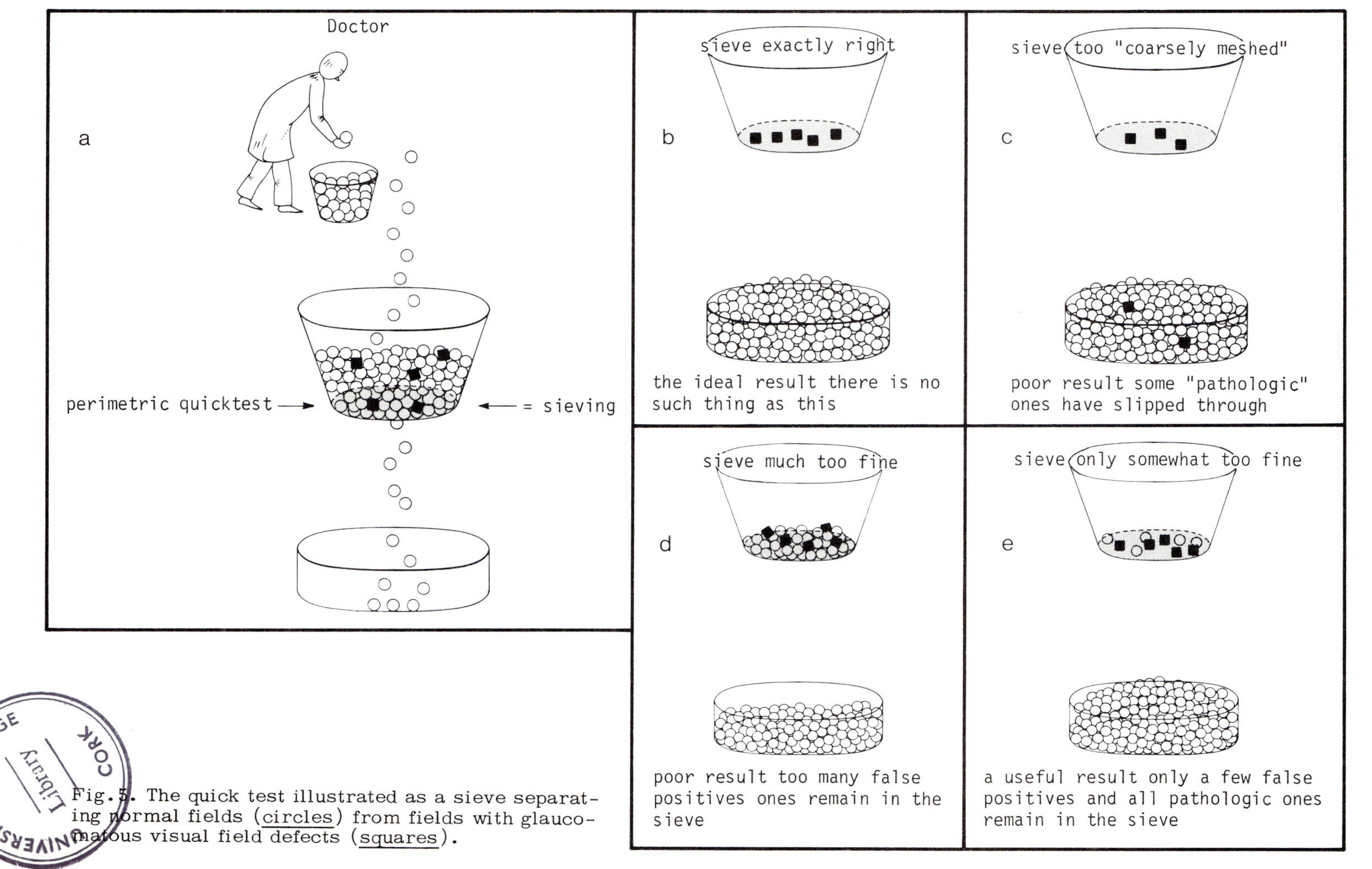

Fig. 5. The quick test illustrated as a sieve separating normal fields (circles) from fields with glaucomatous visual field defects (squares).

of patients would have to be subjected to the lengthy and strenuous process of detailed perimetry.

Such apparently diseased, i.e., false positive, visual field findings can result if too many test points are offered in the quick test, so that the attention of the patient is overtaxed and he responds falsely. Since each examined visual field point is only tested once in the quick test and cannot be checked 'as in usual detailed perimetry' a decrease in the patient's concentration can easily lead to false positive visual fields being found.

HEIJL and KRAKAU and also FRIEDMAN have already chosen the quick test as their examination method. Concerning his test, KRAKAU reports that it lasts only 3 min. This sensationally short time is, however, only bought at the cost of some disadvantages: 9% of the examined patients show a false positive result. The study does not reveal how many false negatives there were, i.e., those that incorrectly appeared as normal visual fields. The authors, however, conclude from the fact that they did not find the blind spot in 11% of the cases that approximately 11% of the small scotomas could also not be found. This is of course a fairly large number and as a result the "sieve" appears to me to be a little too "coarsely meshed."

We have devised a somewhat different quick test plan, which we have built into our automatic Tübingen Perimeter, still under development but already in constant use. This Tübingen quick test is at the moment in the test stage, so that it is as yet too early to make a report of results, but I should like to outline briefly the principle of examination. In this test we have so to speak, deliberately adapted the size of the sieve "mesh" to the size and location of the scotomas of early defects. We have 'in accordance with our conception of a quick test as described above' chosen in preference a "finer-meshed" sieve, so that we can also sift out small scotomas with certainty. The test point is offered in the endangered area at 122 examination points (Fig.6): 116 points serve the purpose of detecting glaucomatous defects, and three on each side are intended additionally for the determination of the blind spot. If the latter is not found, we declare the whole examination invalid, for fixation must then have been so poor that no reliable result can be expected. In this we agree fully with the reflections of BENGTSSON and KRAKAU.

To improve and test the attention of the patient, 12 - 18 pretence test point representations were interspersed in random succession, whereby the patient hears the same sound as he does with genuine test point representations, but where no light in fact appears. At the end of the examination, the computer indicates how often a patient has responded to these pretence representations. If this occurs frequently, the whole result is not evaluated, for the patient's answers are too unreliable; it is then also possible that a response has been made with real scotomas, even though the test point was not seen.

In my opinion, a quick test where the principle is to examine at predetermined, always constant visual field points with a uniform luminance can be used effectively for detecting early defects. It can show whether or not early defects exist. It can, however, give no information concerning the exact extent, form, or depth of the scotomas. It is, however, precisely these three criteria of scotomas that must be known if a statement is to be made as to whether or not a visual field defect increases in the course of disease. In other words, a quick test that examines at fixed points is not suitable for control examinations the purpose of which is to always answer the question concerning progression.

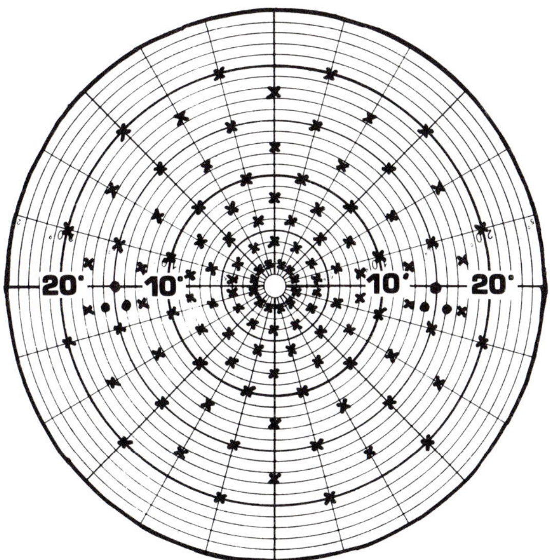

Fig.6. Test points in the Tübinger quick test (crosses). Test points corresponding to the blind spot that will not be detected are presented as closed circles.

I should like to demonstrate this with a short example of a perimetric control examination. An examination along one visual field meridian can give what seems to be a reduction in scotoma size, even though the scotoma has in fact remained the same size in all three examinations. The position of the eye during the process of fixation has only been fixed as regards the horizontal and vertical lines but not regarding rotation around the line of sight as the axis. This can be easily proved by systematic studies on the location of the blind spot in repeated perimetry. The blind spot and scotoma have undergone a slight circular displacement between the first, second, and third examinations. As a result, the meridian examined in the second and third examinations does not run through the middle of the scotoma in the same way as it does the first time. The control examination along the same meridian, therefore, shows changes in the scotoma, which in actual fact do not exist. The examination error described above can only be avoided in perimetry, if the examination points are not fixed rigidly but can be chosen freely during the examination.

However important the development of a good quick test appears to me, it also seems to me to be just as important to attribute to it the function of division into pathologic and healthy visual fields alone, but not to propagate it as the only perimetric method. If we were to do this, the development of the quick test would be synonymous with a step backward in the accuracy of sensory diagnosis.

What I mean, therefore, is that in addition to quick test instruments perimetry must be available, with which visual fields, sifted out as being diseased, can be given a detailed perimetric examination as a basis for later control examinations. With such a combination, first a quick test and then in a pathologic case a detailed perimetric examination, it should be possible 'in my opinion' to not only evaluate correctly the disease of individual patients, but above all to come closer to an understanding of glaucoma disease from a pathophysiologic point of view.

Discussion

ARMALY: I have a few comments on the different presentations.
The first ist that there seems to be a difference between Europe and the United States with regards to the earliest defect in glaucoma or the one that we should detect. We have been pursuing the earliest defect in glaucoma and find it to be a relative, not an absolute, defect and that at this stage some of the defects are reversible. In the collaborative study, we chose to detect the early relative defect by utilizing threshold at 25° from fixation to test the paracentral area in selective perimetry. Because of the possibility of reversibility of the early stage, we should refine our detection to encompass this stage even if that is difficult rather than go after the absolute defect when reversibility is not to be expected. The early stage we should aim for is stage I, not stage II, of Dr. AULHORN, so that our screening method may have false positives but no false negatives.
The second is to welcome the introduction of automated perimetry and its first results as presented by Dr. BENGTSSON. The main advantage as I see it is standardization of the test so that now we can study the physiologic or pathologic variation of the system without the variable performer. We should keep in view the fact that the sensitivity of the system changes and that not all change is performer or instrument error.
The third is to emphasize the need to look for other modalities of visual function that might show an earlier change than perimetric findings: color abnormality, brightness discrimination, etc.

KRIEGLSTEIN: We are running a project on the reproducibility of well-established paracentral field defects using the Goldmann perimeter and the automated perimeter of Krakau. Two observers used both methods under blind conditions. There were many more defects missed using the kinetic perimeter than with the computer perimeter. Therefore, we assume that screening perimetry in glaucoma should be computer-assisted.

BENGTSSON: We are well aware that early visual field defects in glaucoma are variable and sometimes reversible. In fact, the field defect chosen to illustrate the mode of representation in one of my slides could not be confirmed a few weeks after its detection. (Later on, a similar defect reappeared in the same location).
As for the variability of early glaucomatous visual field defects, preliminary data suggest that such variations are more closely associated with changes in the systemic blood pressure than with changes in the ocular tension.
Yet our main concern in automatic perimetry is its specificity. At present, we have found 70 defects at screening. Only 14 (20%) of them were glaucomatous. We are,

therefore, not inclined to believe that (in the terminology of Prof. AULHORN) the "sieve" of our automatic perimeter is too "coarsely meshed."

PODOS: Contrast sensitivity is the inverse of contrast threshold, the ability to see a bar pattern grating at minimal contrast. One varies the contrast and can also test at various widths of the grating. The fewer the bars on the oscilloscope, the lower the spatial frequency. Arden has reported a reduction of contrast sensitivity to stationary patterns of low spatial frequency in glaucoma patients. The pattern can be presented stationary or it can be alternated between light and dark, so-called counterphase presentation. The latter presentation produces a sensitivity curve that at low spatial frequencies rises above the stationary presentation in normal but not glaucoma patients. Drs. ATKINS, BODIS-WOLLNER, WOLKSTEIN, MOSS, and I have tested patients with counterphase flickering gratings of two low spatial frequencies. We looked at 37 normals, 10 ocular hypertensives, and 11 patients with primary open-angle glaucoma. All had at least 20/30 vision. The mean sensitivity of the two measurements was consistently lower in the glaucomatous eyes as compared to the normal eyes (only one exception in each group). It was also reduced in about one-half of the ocular hypertensive eyes although they had normal fields and optic nerve heads. These results could not be accounted for by the medications being used by the patients. A prospective study has been initiated of the ocular hypertensive patients as this test may have prognostic significance.

HARMS: To avoid the influence of rotation, I recommend cheking the position of the blind spot by careful kinetic perimetry and determining the center of the blind spot. When we determine a radial meridian and a circle line through this center by profile perimetry, we then have a "position cross." Before the repetition of perimetry, expecially of profile perimetry, we have to find the position cross of the blind spot. Then we can calculate the rotation, evaluating the results of profile perimetry, assuming control fixation of the patient.

PHELPS: Regarding cyclorotations during perimetry and the effect of those rotations on the reproducibility of profile perimetry, do we have evidence that this varies from day to day? If it does, could it also vary from minute to minute during the examination? Could it be controlled by using a cross rather than a point for fixation?

SHAFFER: How quick is the quick test?"

AULHORN: Five minutes.

DRANCE: I agree completely with Dr. ARMALY that our screening must aim at relative not absolute scotoma. In the cases I showed of the paracentral scotoma that occurred in patients with a previously normal visual field, eight of the nine were in fact relative. Any screening procedure should have false positives, otherwise it misses many defects.

GREVE: It seems to be agreed upon that we have to separate a detection phase from a second phase, which I have called assessment phase. The requirements for both phases are different. There also seems to be agreement that in the detection phase a grid of evenly distributed static stimuli is to used, with the exception of the periphery. Thirdly, we agree that this grid of stimuli should not be used for the assessment of defects and its subsequent follow-up. This means that instruments like the visual field analyzer and Krakau-Heijl's automatic caompimeter are basically detection instruments and are not suitable for follow-up studies.
The normal variation is in the order of 0.3 log units. Pathologic variation in permetric defects is considerably larger. These types of variation have to be differentiated. Early defects have to exceed the pathologic variation.
We have described the early defects as relative defects with an intensity of or at least 0.5 log units and a width of at least 3^{0} in the upper part and preferably demonstrable in adjacent meridians, that is, in the course of the nerve fiber bundles. These wedge-shaped defects may go through a fluctuation stage before they develop into defects for maximum luminance. This stage of a fluctuating defect may be of interest for therapeutic decisions. It is the only stage where reversibility is seen frequently.
We have to program our detection methods in such a way that these early fluctuating defects can be found.
We have to abandon the idea that visual field examination is a quick, cheap, and easy procedure. Only the detection procedure can be relatively quick; the assessment phase that starts once a defect has been found is unfortunately time-consuming, requires excellently trained personnel, and good instruments.

AULHORN: Closing remarks

1) To Dr. GREVE:
I am pleased that you agree concerning my view that a perimetric quick test (with a limited number of test spots) is only useful for detection but not for follow-up of early glaucomatous visual field defects.

2) To Dr. SHAFFER:
The examination with one light intensity of the test spot takes approximately 5 min. Experience must show whether we need one intensity of the test spot or more.

3) To Dr. ARMALY and Dr. DRANCE:

Even in Europe, the earliest visual field defects in glaucoma are relative. Only those defects are reversible in my view. The first relative stage proceeds early to the second with absolute scotomata in our belief.

Since a relative scotoma might be too small to be differentiated from physiologic variability, I cannot believe that a quick test will in any case detect a relative defect with certainty. Relative visual field defects with severely raised thresholds will certainly be detected with a quick test if we use a lower rather than the higher intensity of the test spot. Our prototype of such a machinery works with two different intensities (32 and 3.2 cd/m^2). Experience must show whether this is sufficient or not.

Every quick test is a compromise. If we do not spend the time on an extensive examination, we should use the limited examination time for checking a large number of test spot locations instead of a few test spot locations but many test spot intensities. This decreases the risk of missing a visual field defect in our opinion.

4) To Dr. PHELPS:

In general, we notice no cyclorotation in the course of a perimetric examination as evidenced by perimetry of the blind spot at the beginning and end of the examination. There are no reports of whether a cross as a fixational object will inhibit cyclo rotation. In our view, the form of the fixation point exerts no influence on cyclorotation.

5) To Dr. BENGTSSON:

Every examination with prefixed test spots will be too coarsely meshed since the early visual field defects have an extension of only a few degrees and appear in every position of the central visual field. The probability of detection of a visual field defect is increased by the number of test spots. Our number of test spots is still a coarsely meshed grid, which means a compromise. The more the better!

Autoregulation of Blood Flow in the Distal Segment of the Optic Nerve*

J. Terry Ernest

University of Wisconsin Hospitals, Center for Health Sciences, 1300 University Ave., Madison, Wisc. 53706, USA

Autoregulation of blood flow may be defined as the adjustment of blood flow through an organ to provide for its metabolic needs. Autoregulation is a part of homeostasis, which is the more general term for the stability in the internal environment achieved by control mechanisms activated by negative feedback. It is usually thought of in a relatively restricted sense as the intrinsic tendency of an organ to maintain constant blood flow despite changes in perfusion pressure (13). Vascular tone and its control is under the influence of neurogenic and hormonal factors, but autoregulatory mechanisms operate at the local level. The autoregulatory mechanisms may be influenced and even overridden by nervous and blood factors, but they operate even if sympathectomy is carried out and catecholamines are excluded.

The local factors responsible for autoregulation are poorly understood. It appears that the smooth muscle coats of arteries have an inherent tendency to constrict when the blood pressure increases so that the capillaries are essentially protected from the pressure elevations. This can be demonstrated in the circulation of the eye by occluding a retinal vein. Obstruction of a retinal vein results in an elevation of the peripheral resistance and thus raises the blood pressure in the capillaries and arteries, which is followed by an immediate constriction of the arteries (2). On the other hand, a local increase in tissue metabolites has a vasodilator action, which can also be demonstrated in the retinal circulation. If the retina is made ischemic by induced elevation of the intraocular pressure, the retinal arteries are seen to dilate when the pressure is normalized (ERNEST, unpublished). The retinal circulation autoregulates, and it is generally accepted that the choroidal circulation, at least in the physiologic range, does not. (1, 12, 15) It is of some importance to understand the normal regulation of the blood flow of the distal segment of the optic

---

* This study was supported in part by US Public Health Service Research Grant EV 02526 and a Research to Prevent Blindness, Inc., Eye Research Professorship.

nerve because if it responds passively to changes in the perfusion pressure, optic nerve damage in glaucoma is easy to understand. However, if the optic disk circulation autoregulates, the effects of elevated intraocular pressures become exceedingly complex. If the latter is true, then we must study the mechanisms of autoregulation to learn why, in chronic open-angle glaucoma after a period of years at intraocular pressures that can be compensated by adjustments in the circulation, there is an eventual failure of the mechanisms.

Local Temperature as a Measure of Blood Flow

The amount of heat produced by the tissue of the distal segment of the optic nerve is negligible in comparison with the heat transferred to it by the blood. The optic disk, however, constantly loses heat to the vitreous, and in fact there is a gradient of heat loss from posterior to anterior in the eye (14). Thus, changes in the local blood flow of the optic disk will result in changes in the temperature of the tissue. Therefore, relative changes in the blood flow of the optic nerve can be monitored with a thermocouple (10). A refinement of the technique is to add a heating element to the tissue to increase the measured temperature gradient (3). The techniques are, of course, invasive and have only been used in cats and monkeys. The results, however, are of interest since they suggest that both the blood vessels on the surface of the optic disk and those 2 - 4 mm behind the lamina cribrosa autoregulate. When the intraocular pressure was elevated and then rapidly returned to normal, optic disk surface temperature overshot the baseline level indicating the vessels had begun to compensate for the abnormal intraocular pressure. Optic nerve temperature measurements behind the lamina cribrosa showed little change until the intraocular pressure had exceeded 50 mmHg, indicating that the circulation was initially able to compensate for the elevated intraocular pressure by autoregulating.

Tissue Oxygen Tension Measurement

Tissue oxygen tensions may be measured in vivo by using a platinum microelectrode to electrolyze the dissolved oxygen. The extracellular microelectrodes are polarized with a voltage of 0.6 and oxygen is then the only reducible substance (6). Tissue oxygen tension measurements have been made on the surface of the optic disk in cats and in the prelaminar optic disk area of rhesus monkeys (7, 9). In the latter studies, the central retinal artery was interrupted to prevent confounding the results by the normal oxygen leakage from the large vessel. A decrease in the perfusion pressure, accomplished by either increasing the intraocular pressure or by decreasing cardiac output, resulted in a transient decrease in tissue oxygen tensions followed by recovery to baseline levels within approximately 90 s.

Tissue oxygen tensions depend on blood flow and to some extent on extraction of oxygen from the blood as well as cellular utilization. A more efficient distribution of the local blood flow might also change tissue oxygen tension, but optic nerve capillaries are probably similar to those of brain and retina, which do not normally have segmental areas of capillary nonperfusion. Tissue oxygen tensions measured in the capillary-free fovea centralis, which reflect choroidal blood flow, do not autoregulate (11). This suggests that the optic disk measurements are due to local circulatory adaptation. The optic disk oxygen tension recovery following a decrease in perfusion pressure was eliminated by hypercapnia. This is evidence that the process is due to autoregulation of the circulation on the surface and in the prelaminar areas of the optic disk.

Blood Flow Measurement by Hydrogen Clearance

The clearance or desaturation of tissues that have been saturated with highly diffusable gases reflects the local blood flow (4). A number of assumptions must be made, but if the central retinal artery is interrupted, the technique may be employed to measure blood flow in the prelaminar area of the optic disk (8). Platinum microelectrodes, similar to those used in the tissue oxygen measurement studies, are inserted into the tissue of the optic disk. The microelectrodes must be plated with palladium and polarized with a voltage of 0.3. The animals are saturated by the inhalation of 4% hydrogen gas; the gas is turned off, the desaturation curve recorded, and its half-time measured. Since hydrogen gas is inert and freely diffusable, its removal from the tissue depends on the local blood flow.

These blood flow studies were carried out on rhesus monkeys who had their intraocular pressures artificially regulated. Blood flow in the prelaminar area of the optic disk autoregulated over a wide range of intraocular pressures. Moreover, if the intraocular pressure was rapidly returned to normal following several minutes of elevation, there was a transient overshoot with a blood flow greater than normal. This is further evidence of autoregulation of the circulation in the prelaminar area of the optic nerve.

Blood Flow Measurement by Microspheres

Microspheres, injected into the left heart, may be used to study the fractional distribution of blood flow to local vascular beds. This is based on the assumption that the microspheres are well-mixed, are distributed in proportion to blood flow, are impacted in the capillaries of the tissue without affecting the blood flow, and do not escape to the venous circulation and recirculate (15). Recently, BILL and GEIJER (5) reported a study in which they measured the number of microspheres impacted following their injection in monkeys by counting them in serial sections of the distal segment of the optic nerve. The investigators compared eyes with elevated intraocular pressures with their fellow normal eyes and found autoregulation of the circulation in the prelaminar area of the optic nerve. It is interesting to note that there was an increase in blood flow in the retrolaminar area of the optic nerve with elevations in the intraocular pressure that was not observed in the studies employing the heated thermocouple technique (3).

Discussion

The studies herein reviewed have all been, to one degree or another, invasive. The most serious criticism, however, is the fact that the work was carried out on young, healthy animals. Even if one overlooks the problem of extrapolating data obtained from animals to humans, chronic open-angle glaucoma is a disease of middle age. Nonetheless, there is considerable evidence that the blood flow of the distal segment of the optic nerve autoregulates. Moreover, the circulation is apparently able to compensate for elevations in the intraocular pressure well within the range of chronic open-angle glaucoma. We are left with concluding that either glaucomatous optic nerve disease is not due to a compromise of the optic disk circulation or else there is an eventual breakdown in the autoregulatory mechanisms that normally keep the blood flow at levels adequate for the requirements of the tissue. If the latter is the case, perhaps the most urgent need is for the development of methods of assessing the competency and the reserve of the autoregulatory mechanisms so we can predict which patients are destined to develop loss of tissue and impairment of visual functions.

Summary

Microelectrodes are used to measure optic disk and optic nerve temperature, oxygen tension, and hydrogen clearance all believed to reflect blood flow. Using these and other techniques, it has been shown that experimental elevations of the intraocular pressure of the same order of magnitude as are associated with chronic open-angle glaucoma have little effect on optic nerve blood flow. Thus, the blood flow of the distal segment of the optic nerve autoregulates. Autoregulation is defined as the intrinsic tendency of an organ to maintain constant blood flow despite changes in perfusion pressure. The conclusion is that either glaucomatous optic nerve disease is not due to a compromise of the optic disk circulation or else there is an eventual breakdown in the autoregulatory mechanisms that normally keep the blood flow at levels adequate for the requirements of the tissue.

References

(1) Alm, A.; Bill, A.: The oxygen supply to the retina. II. Effects of high intraocular pressure and of increased arterial carbon dioxide tension on uveal and retinal blood flow in cats. Acta Physiol. Scand. 84, 306-319 (1972)

(2) Archer, D.B.; Ernest, J.T.; Maguire, C.J.F.: Experimental branch retinal vein obstruction. In: Vision and circulation. 3rd William Mackenzie Symposium. Cant. J. S. (ed.) pp. 226-242. Saint Louis: Mosby 1976

(3) Armaly, M.F.; Araki, M.: Optic nerve circulation and ocular pressure. Invest. Ophthalmol. 14, 724-731 (1975)

(4) Aukland, K.; Bower, B.R.; Berliner, R.W.: Measurement of local blood flow with hydrogen gas. Circ. Res. 14, 164-187 (1964)

(5) Bill, A.; Geijer, C.: Effect of intraocular pressure on regional blood flow in the retina and optic nerve. Association for Research in Vision and Ophthalmology Spring Meeting. Sarasota (Florida), 1977

(6) Ernest, J.T.: In vivo measurement of optic disk oxygen tension. Invest. Ophthalmol. 12, 927-931 (1973)

(7) Ernest, J.T.: Autoregulation of optic disk oxygen tension. Invest. Ophthalmol. 13, 101-106 (1974)

(8) Ernest, J.T.: Optic disk blood flow. Trans. Ophthalmol. Soc. U.K. 96, 348-351 (1976)

(9) Ernest, J.T.: Optic disk oxygen tension. Exp. Eye Res. 24, 271-278 (1977)

(10) Ernest, J.T.; Potts, A.M.: Pathophysiology of the distal portion of the optic nerve. IV. Local temperature as a measure of blood flow. Am. J. Ophthalmol. 72, 435-444 (1971)

(11) Ernest, J.T.; Stern, W.H.; Archer, D.B.: Submacular choroidal circulation. Am. J. Ophthalmol. 81, 574-582 (1976)

(12) Ffytche, T.J.; Bulpitt, C.J.; Kohner, E.M.; Archer, D.; Dollery, C.T.: Effect of changes in intraocular pressure on the retinal microcirculation. J. Ophthalmol. 58, 514-522 (1974)

(13) Johnson, P.C.: Review of previous studies and current theories of autoregulation. Circ. Res. 15, [Suppl. 1] 1-9 (1964)

(14) Schwartz, B.; Feller, M.R.: Temperature gradients in the rabbit eye. Invest. Ophthalmol. 1, 513-521 (1962)

(15) Weiter, J.J.; Schachar, R.A.; Ernest, J.T.: Control of intraocular blood flow. I. Intraocular pressure. Invest. Ophthalmol. 12, 327-331 (1973)

Discussion

BILL: As mentioned by Dr. ERNEST, we have found autoregulation of the blood flow in the prelaminar part of the optic nerve, i.e., a blood flow that is very moderately influenced even by marked variation in perfusion pressure. A reduction in perfusion pressures from the normal level to about 30 mm Hg caused only 20% - 30% reduction in blood flow. In the lamina and just behind, there was no appreciable reduction. These experiments as well as those described by Dr. ERNEST were performed during short periods of intraocular pressure. It seemed possible that autoregulatory mechanisms might last over longer periods of time. We have, therefore, performed some experiments in which the eye pressure was maintained at a high level for 5 - 6 h. The results were very much the same. This result is of considerable interest since it has been shown by Anderson and others that axoplasmic flow is seriously affected at perfusion pressures around 25 - 35 mm Hg.
Axoplasmic flow was more or less stopped within the lamina. It seems that there is a poor correlation between effects on blood flow and axoplasmic flow. It is quite possible that inhomogeneous blood flow within the lamina may result in small regions with poor nutrition in spite of overall normal blood flow. It is certainly possible that this may also occur in chronic open-angle glaucoma, but these phenomena remain to be proved.

DRANCE: Does the homeostatic mechanism change with chronic changes of pressure, particularly in young people?

LEYDHECKER: 1) Is the autoregulation age-dependent?
2) Is any one of your methods to measure blood flow better than the other, in the sense that it shows less standard variation or physiologically more acceptable values?

BENGTSSON: In a survey of 1010 subjects (79% of the population aged 55 - 70 years in a defined area), we found ten simplex glaucomas with the automatic perimeter described by HEIJL and KRAKAU (1975). Seven of those ten simplex glaucomas were low-tension glaucomas (with intraocular pressures consistently below 24.5 mm Hg in both eyes). All seven had optic disk hemorrhages of the kind described by Drance. This finding would suggest a localized breakdown of the autoregulation of blood flow in part of the optic disk as a common cause of damage to the optic nerve fibers in glaucoma simplex.

ERNEST (reply): It is most reasonable to expect that autoregulatory mechanisms are damaged by systemic diseases, especially hypertensive cardiovascular disease, but thus far we do not have any data to support this hypothesis. Similarly, changes due to age with the loss of endothelial and mural cells must result in loss of adaptive function, but experimental studies are lacking because we do not have aged experimental animals and we do not have a clinical test to measure autoregulation in man.

None of the methods of measuring blood flow in the distal segment of the optic nerve are very good because they are invasive. The microsphere method is the least invasive, but the number of spheres injected must be kept as small as possible so that they do not reflect blood flow in a completely impacted vasculature.

Finally, I have defined autoregulation in a very general way to avoid implications about the actual mechanisms because these are so poorly understood. I would like to thank Drs. DRANCE, LEYDHECKER, BENGTSSON, BILL, and LANGHAM for their discussions, and I am grateful to the International Glaucoma Committee for the opportunity to present my paper.

Observer Variation in Applanation Tonometry and Estimation of the Cup Disk Ratio

Wolfgang Leydhecker, Günter K. Krieglstein, E. v. Collani

University, Eye Hospital, Josef-Schneider-Straße 11, D-8700 Würzburg, Germany (FRG)

The aim of the present study was to establish the reproducibility of applanation tonometric results and of the estimation of the cup/disk ratio. The knowledge about the interobserver variation in both parameters is of significance to assess the reliability of the individual finding, because decisions concerning the kind of treatment are dependent thereon. The clinical studies were divided into four groups: the intra- and interobserver variation in tonometry and the intra- and interobserver variation in the estimation of the cup/disk ratio.

Intraobserver Variation in Applanation Tonometry

Methods

To quantitate the intraobserver variation in applanation tonometry, the scale of a Goldmann Tonometer was covered by a small plastic ring, so that the tonometrist could not read the value on the scale corresponding to the steady-state intraocular pressure (IOP). The value given on the scale was read by a technician who stripped off the plastic ring for a second and replaced the scale to zero. This procedure of taking applanation pressures under strictly blind conditions for the observer was maintained throughout the present tonometric studies. Each observer did six applanation readings with a 1-min time interval (controlled by stop watch) in 15 patients. The application of fluorescein and topical anesthetics was up to the observer. There had been nine observers with 1 or 2 years of experience in clinical tonometry, six observers with 3 or 4 years of experience in tonometry, and three observers with more than 10 years of experience. The whole series comprises the results of 270 patients and 1620 applanation readings.

Results

The relative frequency of differences of two subsequent applanation readings in one individual eye by one observer, done under strictly blind conditions, is illustrated in Fig. 1. If we accept a difference of two subsequent applanation readings between

0 and 2 mm Hg as an indication of sufficient reproducibility, 76.5% of the repeated measurements in observer group I, 82.5% of the paired measurements in observer group II, and 82% of the paired measurements in observer group III (experienced ophthalmologists) were valid. The appropriate statistical parameter to describe the intraobserver variation in tonometry is the confidence interval of 90% of paired differences. The confidence interval signifies the range of 90% of the differences (first pressure reading minus second reading) we have to expect. Since the second read-

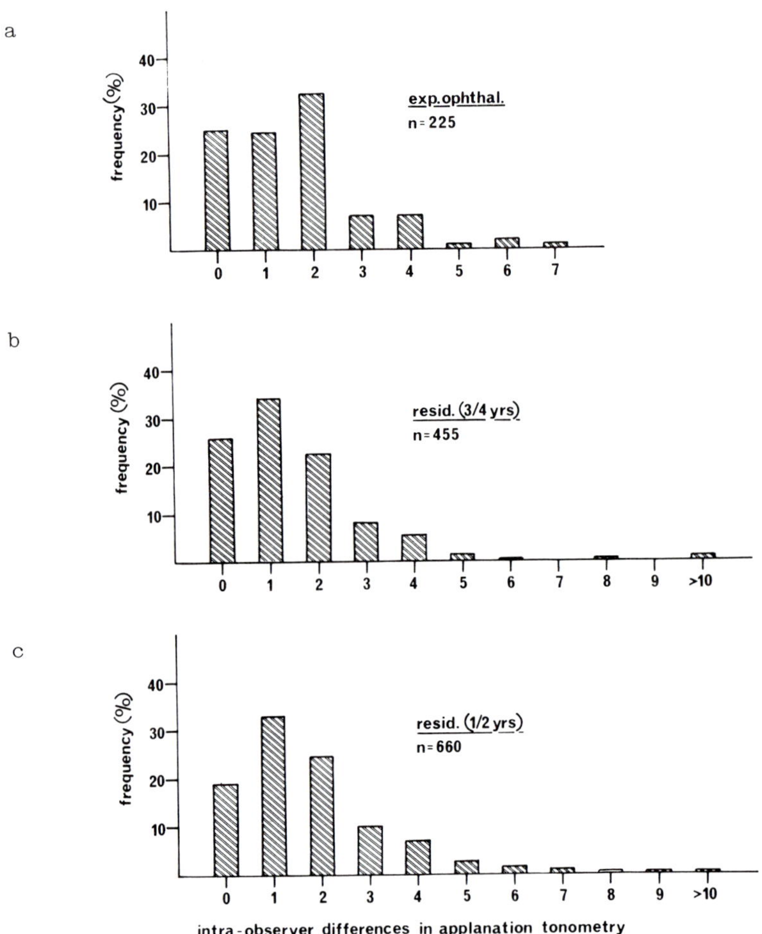

Fig. 1a-c. The frequency distribution of the differences in paired measurements of the IOP. The abscissa shows the magnitude of the differences in subsequent applanation readings done by one observer in one eye. The ordinate gives the relative frequency. a the results for experienced ophthalmologists; b the results for residents with 3 or 4 years training; c the results for residents with 1 or 2 years training.

ing can be either higher or lower than the first reading, the confidence interval is expressed as ±. In that respect, the confidence interval of observer group I was ± 4.57 mm Hg, for observer group II ± 3.75 mm Hg, and for observer group III ± 3.61 mm Hg. There seems to be less scatter in repeated applanation tonometry with increasing experience in tonometric routine. The mean value of differences of paired measurements in observer group I was 1.79 mm Hg, in observer group II 1.51 mm Hg, and in observer group III 1.46 mm Hg. The difference between groups I and II was statistically significant at the 1% level of probability (paired t-test).

If we calculate the differences between two subsequent readings from the first to the sixth applanation reading, we find that the confidence intervals of 90% decrease from 3.86 to 3.23 mm Hg. That means that in the individual eye the reproducibility of tonometric results will improve with repeated tonometry. The largest differences occurred between the first two applanation readings.

If we consider differences not between single values but between mean values of two applanation readings (e.g., mean value of first and second readings compared to mean value of second and third readings) the reproducibility of tonometric results is significantly better. The confidence interval of 90% of these differences between mean values of two readings ranges between ± 2.89 and ± 2.57 mm Hg. Differences between mean values of three applanation readings (first to third readings versus third to sixth readings) have even less confidence intervals (90%), viz., ± 2.11 mm Hg, signifying good reproducibility.

The effect of repeated tonometry in 270 patients was calculated from the mean values and standard errors of the means of all first readings, all second readings, etc. There is a gradual pressure decrease in repeated tonometry as previously described by KRAKAU (1).

Interobserver Variation in Applanation Tonometry

Methods

Fifty-seven patients were investigated in this series. One eye in each patient was measured under blind conditions as previously mentioned by six different observers. Each pressure measurement was separeted by 2 or 3 min, and the patient was moved from one examination room to the next. Application of fluorescein and anesthetics was up to the individual observer.

Results

The frequency distribution of differences of paired measurements of different observers in one individual eye is shown in Fig. 2. Again, if we consider differences of 0 - 2 mm Hg between two and successive readings as an indication of good reproducibility, 63% of the paired measurements are valid. The confidence interval of 90% between two successive readings ranges between ± 5.02 and ± 6.44 mm Hg. The mean value of all paired differences was 2.31 mm Hg. Again, there is a gradual decrease of IOP of about 2 mm Hg over the number of applanation procedures.

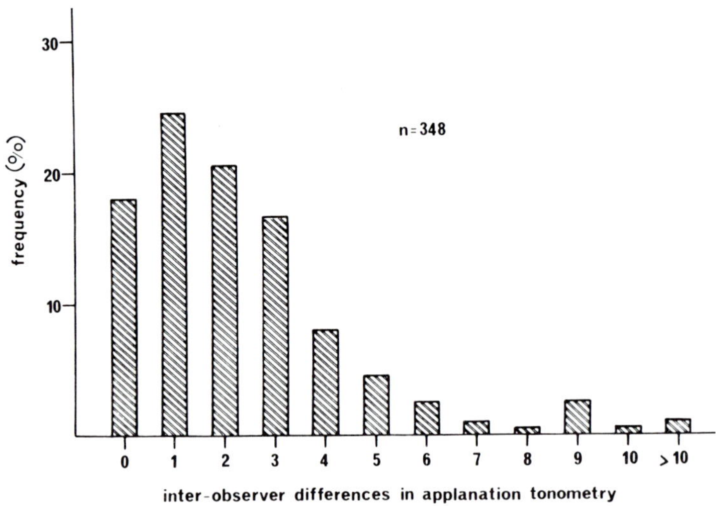

Fig. 2. The relative frequency of differences in paired IOP measurements performed by different observers. The ordinate shows the relative frequency of the differences and the abscissa the magnitude of the differences in subsequent readings. The results are based on 348 comparisons.

Comment

The reasons for the differences in clinical tonometry as described above are the instrument's error, the observer's error, the physiologic variability of IOP and the effect of the tonometric procedure itself on IOP. The instrument's error is fairly low, as we know from calibrating procedures on enucleated human eyes. It is about ± 0.5 mm Hg, making the Goldmann applanation tonometer acceptable as the most precise instrument for measuring IOP. However, in the clinical routine of tonometry, things are different. The observer's technique is quite different, as shown in our series subdivided into three observer groups with different experience. The most relevant reason for differences in tonometric results is the physiologic variability of IOP (2). There are several physiologic influences acting on the IOP, making it a parameter varying within certain ranges. The amplitude of intraocular pulse ranges between 1 mm Hg and 8 mm Hg. In applanation tonometry, the observer has to average the pulsations of the fluorescein semicircles, which can be difficult in pulse amplitudes of more than 5 mm Hg. In longer intervals between repeated pressure measurements, vasomotoric waves of IOP might be superimposed. In pressure measurements done in different examination rooms, the effect of walking obviously influences the IOP. Besides the different physiologic aspects of variability of IOP, the tonometric procedure itself affects the parameter that we want to measure. There had been numerous papers dealing with the effect of repeated tonometry on the IOP, stating unisonally that there is a exponential decrease of IOP over the number of applanations.

Relevance of the Present Results for Clinical Routine

A single IOPD measurement is obviously inadequate for therapeutic decisions or in screening for glaucoma. Our results indicate differences of subsequent tonometries of more than 2 mm Hg in about 20% of the cases. If glaucoma screening is based on a single applanation tonometry, this will imply that this kind of screening will give about 20% false negatives or false positives. PHELPS and PHELPS (4) found in paired measurements using the Goldmann tonometer differences of at least 2 mm Hg in 50% of the eyes tested and 3 mm Hg or more in 30% of the eyes tested. This agrees with our results in interobserver variation. In intraobserver variation, we had significantly less scatter of paired measurements. One cannot give a guideline for optimal tonometry, but if one wishes as much information on IOP one has to focus on mean values of profile tonometry. Despite the decrease of pressure in repeated tonometry, large errors in either direction will be averaged.

Intraobserver Variation in Cup/Disk Ratio Estimation

Methods

Color slides of the optic disks of 50 eyes with intraocular hypertension of 25 patients were presented twice, with a time lapse of 5 weeks, to ten different residents with 1 - 4 years training in ophthalmology. They were asked to estimate the horizontal and vertical cup/disk ratio. The color slides had been obtained at a pupillary diameter of at least 5 mm. The beginning of the slope at the neuroretinal rim had been identified to be the beginning of the cup. Five ophthalmologists with more than 10 years of experience did the same test again with a 5-week time lapse. None of the observers of either group were previously familiar with the disks presented in the slides. There had been seven possibilities to estimate the relative cup diameter: 0.2 or less, 0.3, 0.4, 0.5, 0.6, 0.7, and 0.8 or more.

Results

The relative frequency of the differences in repeated estimation of the vertical and horizontal cup/disk ration in both groups of observers is shown in Fig.3 and 4. If we accept a difference of 0.1 between the first and the second estimations of the cup/disk ratio to represent good reproducibility, the results were as follows. The residents identified the cup/disk ratio in their second estimation with 0.1 differ-

horizontal c/d-ratio

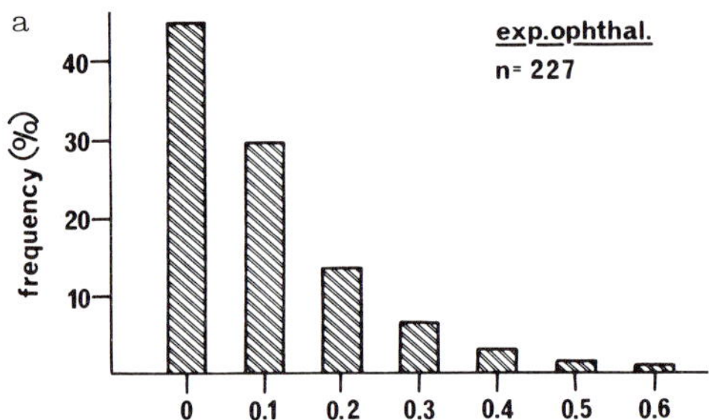

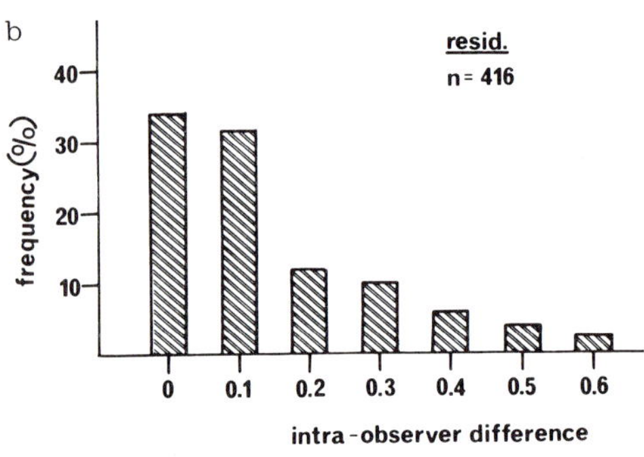

Fig.3, a-b. The frequency distribution of the differences in repeated estimation of the horizontal cup/disk ratio. a the relative frequency of differences in repeated estimation of the horizontal cup/disk ratio for experienced ophthalmologists; b the frequency distribution of the differences for residents.

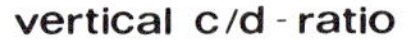

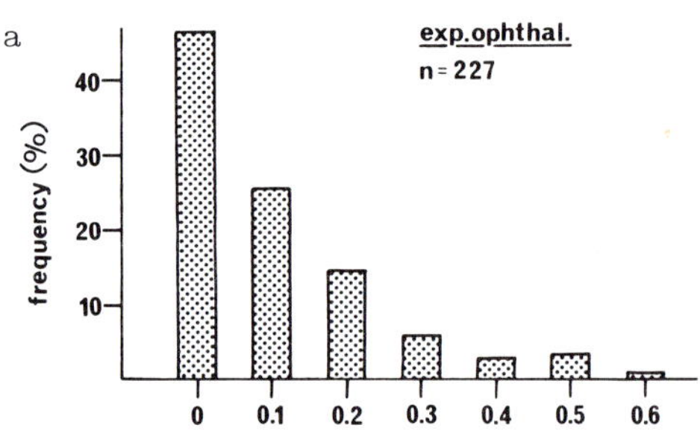

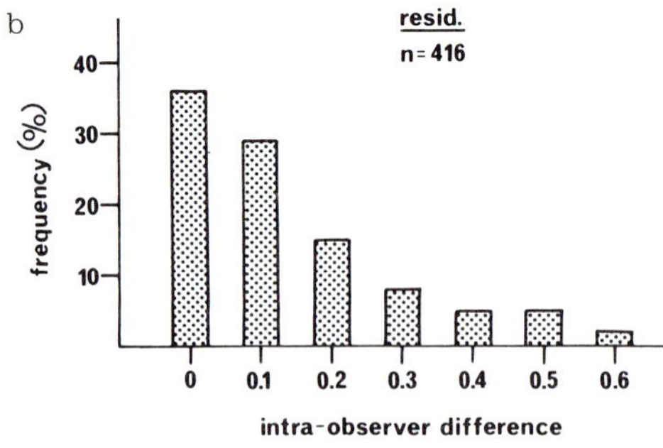

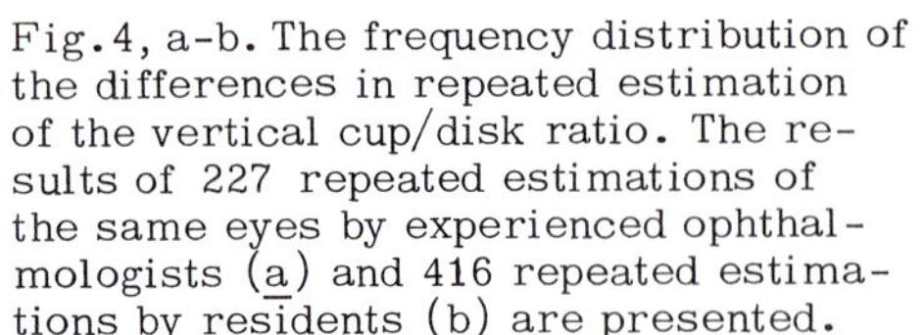

Fig.4, a-b. The frequency distribution of the differences in repeated estimation of the vertical cup/disk ratio. The results of 227 repeated estimations of the same eyes by experienced ophthalmologists (a) and 416 repeated estimations by residents (b) are presented.

ence or less 66% concerning the horizontal and 65% concerning the vertical diameter. The relative frequency of no or only 0.1 difference in repeated estimation in the group of experienced ophthalmologists was 67% in the horizontal and 72% in the vertical diameter. The mean observer difference in the group of residents was 0.15 (horizontal diameter) and 0.15 (vertical diameter). In the group of experienced ophthalmologists, the mean difference of repeated estimation of the cup/disk ratio was 0.12 (horizontal diameter) and 0.13 (vertical diameter). However, intraobserver variations of as much as 0.3 between the first and second estimations were noted even in the group of experienced ophthalmologists with 10 or more years training in approximately 5% and differences of 0.2 were estimated at 13%.

Interobserver Variation in Cup/Disk Ratio Estimation

Methods

The interobserver variation in the cup/disk ratio estimation in 50 ocular hypertensive or glaucomatous eyes of 25 patients, the same subjects as in the clinical studies above, was investigated in the following way. After discontinuation of any local antiglaucomatous treatment and any drug affecting pupillary diameter, 48 h prior to the test, the cup/disk ratio of the horizontal and vertical diameters were estimated by ten different residents with 1 - 4 years training by indirect ophthalmoscopy with a narrow pupil, by direct ophthalmoscopy with the pupil dilated to at least 5 mm, and by stereoscopic contact lens ophthalmoscopy with a dilated pupil.

Results

The relative frequence of the differences in cup/disk ratio estimations of horizontal and vertical diameters between two observers (ten different residents) is shown in Fig. 5 and 6. Both Figures show the results based on three different methods of fundus examination. Differences of 0.1 or less between cup/disk ratio estimation in two observers occurred in 55% of the cases concerning the horizontal diameter and 56% concerning the vertical diameter, when performing indirect ophthalmoscopy with a narrow pupil. Using direct ophthalmoscopy with the pupil dilated, the frequency of a difference of 0.1 or less increased to 65% on the horizontal and 63% on the vertical diameter. Reproducibility of cup/disk ratio estimation between different observers further improved using stereoscopic contact lens ophthalmoscopy. A difference of 0.1 or less occurred in 70% concerning the horizontal diameter and 74.5% concerning the vertical diameter. The reproducibility of cup/disk ratio estimation improved with the quality of fundus examination. The mean values of all cup/disk examinations for the three different methods of ophthalmoscopy are shown in Fig. 7. There is a significant increase in the estimation of the magnitude of the cup diameter from indirect ophthalmoscopy to direct ophthalmoscopy and again to stereoscopic contact lens ophthalmoscopy. Obviously, using indirect ophthalmoscopy in the nondi-

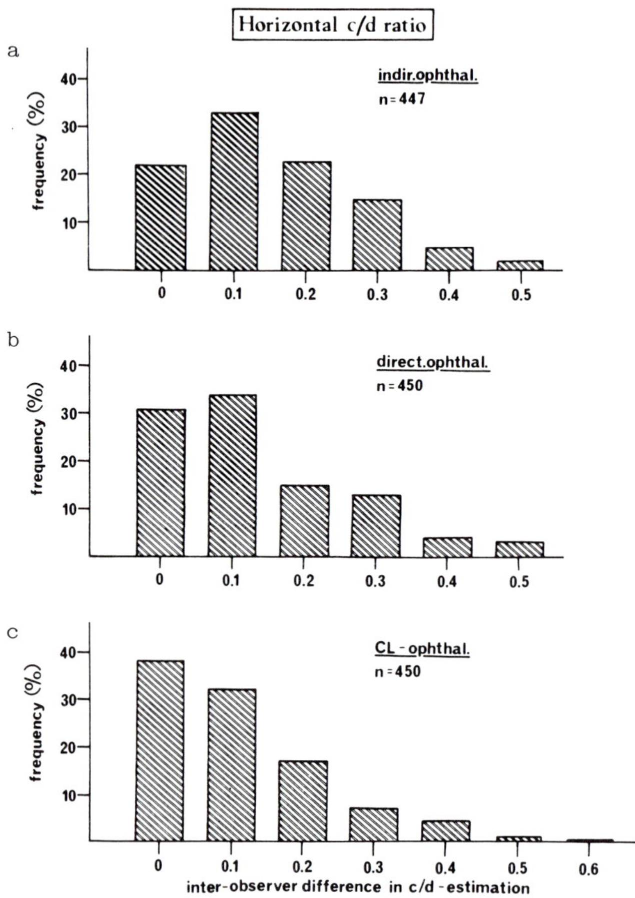

Fig.5, a-c. The frequency distribution of the differences for different observers in horizontal cup/disk ratio estimation. The results of indirect ophthalmoscopy (a), direct ophthalmoscopy (b), and contact lens ophthalmoscopy (c) are presented. The ordinate shows the relative frequency and the abscissa the magnitude of the interobserver differences in cup/disk ratio estimation.

lated pupil and using a monocular examination method, one tends to underestimate the cup size. The statement applies for the horizontal as well as for the vertical cup/disk ratio. The mean difference between two independent observers estimating the horizontal or the vertical cup/disk ratio in an individual eye dependent on different methods of ophthalmoscopy is shown in Fig.8. The mean interobserver variation is fairly large in indirect ophthalmoscopy and lowest in stereoscopic contact lens ophthalmoscopy. The difference in mean values is statistically significant at a 1% level of probability (paired t-test).

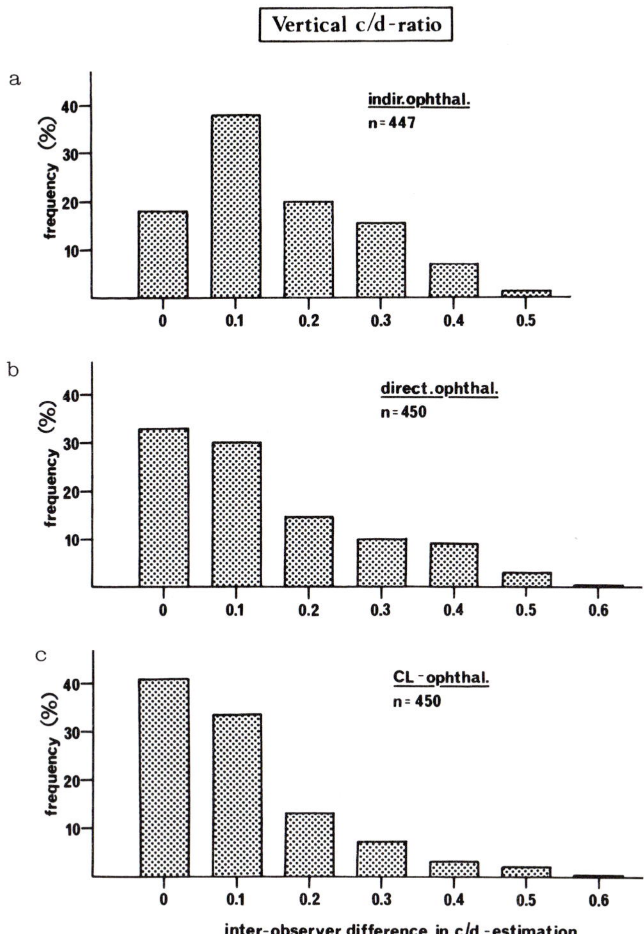

Fig.6, a-c. The frequency distribution of the differences for different observers in vertical cup/disk ratio estimation. The results of indirect ophthalmoscopy (a), direct ophthalmoscopy (b), and contact lens ophthalmoscopy (c) are presented. The ordinate shows the relative frequency and the abscissa the magnitude of the interobserver differences in cup/disk ratio estimation.

Comment

There is no doubt that the estimation of the cup/disk ratio in the horizontal and vertical diameters is just a rough classification of the glaucomatous disk. Consideration of rim notches and the area of pallor or peripapillar hemmorrhages is also very important. However, in clinical routine, disk evaluation is primarily based on the cup/ disk ratio. The present study shows that the reproducibility of the estimation of this parameter is sufficient only under stereoscopic examination conditions. The intra- and interobserver differences of 0.2 that occurred in at least 13% of all tests show that this estimate is rather vague. A cup/disk ratio of 0.3 stands for a normal eye,

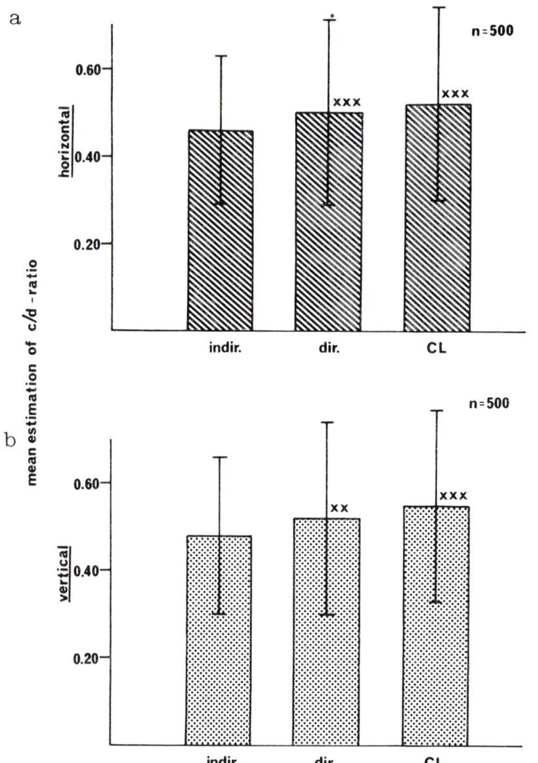

Fig.7, a-b. The mean estimation of the cup/disk ratio in different methods of ophthalmoscopy concerning the horizontal (a) and vertical (b) cup/disk ratio. The difference in mean values of both diameters of cup/disk ratio derived from direct ophthalmoscopy and contact lens ophthalmoscopy is statistically significant from the results derived from indirect ophthalmoscopy at the level of 1% and 0.1% probability (xx, 1% probability of error; xxx, 0,1% probability of error).

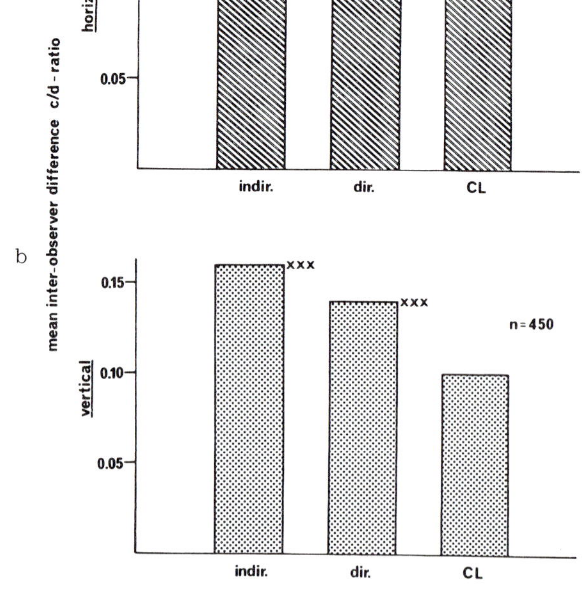

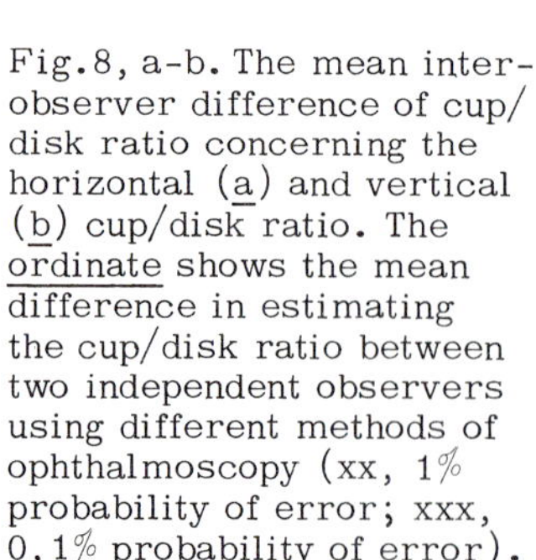
Fig.8, a-b. The mean inter-observer difference of cup/disk ratio concerning the horizontal (a) and vertical (b) cup/disk ratio. The ordinate shows the mean difference in estimating the cup/disk ratio between two independent observers using different methods of ophthalmoscopy (xx, 1% probability of error; xxx, 0,1% probability of error).

whereas 0.5 might already signal early glaucoma. The interobserver variation in cup/disk ratio estimation in screening for glaucoma was intensively investigated (3). The percent of patients reported to have a horizontal cup/disk ratio by LICHTER of less than 0.3 varied from 33% - 72% in five independent examiners. The evaluation of cup/disk ratios from stereoscopic photographs of two eyes by ten expert observers gave a range of individual readings between 0.2 and 0.8 in one eye and in 0.5 and 0.9 in the other eye. This study supports the observation that there is large variability in cup/disk ratio examination as emphasized in our series. The consequence of the present results is to use stereoscopic examination, which minimizes the observer variation, or to make stereoscopic color slides. Simultaneous comparison of stereoscopic slides might provide the highest probability for detecting small differences in the anatomy of the glaucomatous disk.

References

(1) Krakau, C.E.T.; Wilke, K.: On repeated tonometry. Acta Ophthalmol. 49, 611 (1971)

(2) Leydhecker, W.: The intraocular pressure. Clinical aspects. Ann. Ophthalmol. 8, 389 (1976)

(3) Lichter, P.R.: Variability of expert observers in evaluating the optic disk. Trans. Am. Ophthalmol. Soc. 84, 532 (1976)

(4) Phelps, C.D.; Phelps, G.K.: Measurement of intraocular pressure. A study of its reproducibility. Albrecht von Graefes Arch. Ophthalmol. 198, 39 (1976)

Discussion

BENGTSSON: In normal eyes, cup diameters (and cup/disk ratios) are widely dispersed, unevely distributed, and heavily dependent on disk size. "Average rim breadths," on the other hand, are much less dispersed, normally distributed, and independent of the disk diameter. To arrive at a measurement of the average rim breadth, one has to substract the average cup diameter from the average disk diameter. Direct measurements of the rim breadth are useless since the cup seems to "float" around in normal disk (when different disk are compared to each other). The distribution of such measurements is therefore even worse than that of cup diameters.

LEYDHECKER: Could we discuss what in your opinion is more adequate: to note the beginning of the slope or the depth of the excavation that is identical with the area of pallor? Which of these two parameters should we call the cup/disk ratio?

LICHTER: Drs. LEYDHECKER and KRIEGLSTEIN have presented an excellent paper. I would like to show two slides to help make a point. (Slides of both optic disks from a single patient were now shown and the audience asked to commit themselves as to cup/disk ratio and whether the disk was normal or not. There was moderate variability in opinion in cup/disk ratio estimations and the state of normalcy of the disk. However, when the disks were shown side by side rather than separately, the differences in opinion were less). Both of these disks have shown that this expert audience differs in cup/disk ratio estimation. Also shown is the fact that the ratio, by itself, tells us nothing about whether the disk is normal or not.
Measurments of anything imply accuracy and often finality. However, in cup/disk ratio estimation, this is clearly not the case. Both the paper by Profs. LEYDHECKER and KRIEGLSTEIN as well as an exhibit of ours (1) and a subsequent publication (2) showed this. Our own study not only evaluated the variability of experts in determining the cup/disk ratio but also whether the disk was physiologic or pahtologic. We found variability in both parameters. Of course, this study was only designed to test variability in disk evaluation. Once the examiner has the patient before him, looking at both disks, knowing the fields and the pressure, it is far easier to assess the disk correctly. The cup/disk ratio is merely a descriptive term. The higher the cup/disk ratio, the greater the chance that the disk is abnormal.
There are, however, a multitude of configurations the disk can take. For example, a disk with a cup/disk ratio of 0.5 or 0.8 could either be normal, questionable, or abnormal. Thus, while the cup/disk ratio gives some information, the many other factors of the disk that determine whether the disk is normal or not are far more important.

The cup/disk ratio as described by Armaly was not intended to indicate whether the disk was normal or not. However, the popularity of this measurement leads many clinicians to feel that once the number has been recorded, nothing more needs to be done in evaluating the disk. Nothing could be further from the truth.
Perhaps it would be helpful if the International Glaucoma Commitee could agree that the cup/disk ratio is only one of many points to consider and record in optic disk evaluation and that clinicians be encouraged to evaluate the entire disk carefully and to record specifics of their disk findings along with a commitment as to whether the disk looks normal or not.

ARMALY: In Würzberg and Albi, I reported on measurements from stereophotographs of the disk, the cup contour or cup pallor in normal eyes and in eyes with open-angle glaucoma. The results showed clearly that cupping by contour is greater in glaucoma as was the area of pallor. The rim measurement in glaucoma (by subtraction) showed that in glaucoma the rim is thinner in all meridians but thinnest at 6 o'clock and in the oblique meridians, i.e., corresponding to the area of greatest frequency of absolute scotoma. It is important to point out that while we speak of a neuroretinal rim, we have no idea how this is defined nor how variable the estimate is.
Every measurement has a range of variation, and a subjective estimate is more proof of this variation. Nevertheless, proper use of a subjective estimate can be very valuable. It also improves greatly the detection of early glaucoma because of the increasing frequency when the cup/disk ratio is greater than 0.3. To estimate a number is better than verbal description or memory especially for future follow-up. Deep concern about accuracy is influenced greatly by what will happen if we err a little. The answer is nothing terribly important because all it does is increase suspicion.
When I first described this at the academy, I emphasized the variability of this estimate and the importance of recording not only the cup/disk ratio of contour but also of pallor. In addition, I emphasized the need to record as many attributes of the disk blood vessel course as possible because any change is most important clinically. Stereophotography is indeed the best method.
Fortunately, we do not make clinical judgments based on a photograph but evaluate the entire clinical picture and obtain more clues and information that guide clinical judgment.
The contour of the cup and the diameter of pallor are very highly correlated in the normal eye. This is not the case in glaucoma - contour may increase or pallor may increase and we should estimate both from a clinical point of view.
I have two questions. (1) Have you done any measurement in your study on enucleated human eyes to additionally confirm the accuracy of the Goldmann applanation tonome-

ter and have you used this to isolate the former differences? (2) You brought the scale back to zero after each measurement. Every experienced tonometrist can use his own manual sensitivity to turn the drum a given amount. This will tend to reduce intraperformer variation. Why not bring the scale back to our up to an unknown position so that the influence of proprioceptive clues is controlled? Goldmann was against using zero as a starting point because of the undesirable vibrations and recommends ten as the premeasurement position. What is the advantage of zero?

KOLKER: One may estimate the degree of cupping either by measurement of the pallor or the contour. A diagram may be made or estimates of the diameter used as a cup/disk ratio. I have found it most useful to record cup/disk ratios using both factors and indicate "contourcup" and "pallor cup" for each optic disk evaluated. Furthermore, a change may occur in one measurement without a change in the other (and may occur in the absence of and before a change in the visual field). For example, one may note an increase in the "pallor cup" measurement, while the "contour cup" remains unchanged. Similarly, the physical size of the cup (contour) may increase in the absence of any pallor change. Both measurements, therefore, appear to be important.

SHAFFER: In describing the disk, it is important to note the pinkness of the rim in relation to the pallor of the lamina and, secondly, the slope of the rim fibers as they rise toward the retinal level. The rim is the important factor, so my cup/disk ratio as a number is a pallor-to-pinkness ratio. I suggest using a diagram that can indicate pallor-to-pinkness, slope, and irregularities of the rim. This is recorded on a grid divided into 0.2 divisions. It is helpful for those who have no access to stereoscopic photography.

AULHORN: We know that the first visual field defects are located superiorly and inferiorly in the Bjerrum area. These areas belong to the superior and inferior parts of the temporal portion of the disk. Therefore, I think the cup should be measured in the two oblique meridians of the disk. The probability of finding the first pathologic change in the cup should be higher there than in measuring the horizontal and vertical meridians.

HERSCHLER: I would like to call attention to the rim tissue and not the cup. If one ignores the cup and draws the outline and color of the remaining rim tissue, a different picture of the disk will emerge. Local notching and/or hemorrhages will not be missed, and early glaucomatous damage will be detected more rapidly.

DRANCE: The cup/disk ratio and the pallor-to-disc ratio are different measurements and have different meaning. If they are both recorded, the observer becomes aware of that difference. The computer picks both of these and weighs them by separating disks with and without field defects. Other factors such as neuroretinal rim abnormalities, baring of the lamina cribrosa, and hemorrhages at the disk are also picked by the computer in providing more information.

HARMS: One year ago GOLDMANN published a new method for following up any changes in the disk. He photographs the disk and after some time repeats the photograph of the same disk. Then he looks at both pictures through a stereoscope. If a change in the cup occurred during the observation time, we have a stereoscopic effect. I think it is a very simple and ingenious idea. But the observer must have an exact technical method and an excellent stereoscopic vision.

RECCA: I congratulate the authors on their interesting work. It is very important to study the optical disk and measure its variations. I use a method described at the Panamerican meeting in Huston (1972) and in the Symposium of Foz de Iguazu (1974). It is done with the grid ophthalmoscope (Welch-Allyn). We study the temporal rim and measure it. We find that its pathologic variations are in the sector in relation to the arcuate scotoma. In these cases the optic disk can be normal in its other parameters. It is very useful to suspect a glaucoma even in such cases where the intraocular pressure is normal at the time of examination.

SAMPAOLESI: I agree with Dr. AULHORN that it is very important to measure the rim at oblique meridians: temporal, superior, and inferior. We learned from BUSSACCA to measure the rim at these places, with the Goldmann-Bussacca Contact Lens. With such an optical section, we have more and exact information. We note the cup/disk ratio, the pallor, and the width of the temporal rim at different places.
In relation to the interobserver variation of tonometry, we prefer to perform a diurnal pressure curve. When the mean ($\bar{x}$) is more than 19 mm Hg or the diurnal variation is more than 2.8 mm Hg, we consider this a suspect patient, and we make a more frequent control of his pressure.

LEYDHECKER (closing remarks): Thank you for the discussions. It is evident that several different parameters of the optic disk should be noted, such as the beginning of the slope, the area of pallor notching of the rim, hemorrhages, areas of pallor of the rim, and it is also evident that the oblique-vertical diameter is more important than the straight vertical diameter or the horizontal diameter. In our study we took the horizontal and the vertical diameter, not because we thought that these are the most important aspects of the disk but because we felt that for a study of interobserver variation these two parameters could be most easily described to a group.

As to Dr. ARMALY's questions, we have not done measurements on enucleated eyes. I agree that it would be wiser to put the scale back to 10 mm Hg to avoid vibrations, but an examiner tested under blind conditions and knowing that the scale is set at 10 mm Hg would be in a similar advantageous position to feel how much he turns the scale with each measurement, just as when the scale is set at 0.

Important features of the discussions seemed to me that there is no unanimous agreement as to how the cup/disk ratio could be described, whether the cup is measured from the beginning of the slope or at the bottom of the excavation. Disagreement on this question of course, changes completely the significance of any statement on the cup/disk ratio. It should be noted that in the discussion there was a certain evasiveness in giving a special significance to any cup/disk ratio. Evidently, after giving up magic numbers of pressure, we are also giving up magic numbers of cup/disk ratio. We should be careful not to loose our sense for numbers completely. I admit, however, that parameters such as notching of the rim or pallor are difficult to describe in terms of numbers.

I am glad that this group feels what we also showed in our paper, that indirect ophthalmoscopy is not a good method for forming an opinion on the optic disk and that direct ophthalmoscopy is more adequate. If the disk appears suspicious or if there is any reason for a closer examination of the disk, a stereoscopic examination with a dilated pupil should follow with the slit-lamp. The disk examination is just one parameter only, which has its significance in contact with the examination of the second eye, with a study of the visual fields, and with tonometry. The significance of the isolated parameter of disk description has been overemphasized in the last years in my opinion. Disk changes are an event secondary to pressure changes. A careful registration of intraocular pressure and visual fields are in my opinion at least as important as the registration of disk changes. It will show an earlier phase of damage, while the disk atrophy shows the partial death of the optic nerve. We here to act befor this death occurs.

Pathogenesis of Block of Rapid Orthograde Axonal Transport by Elevated Intraocular Pressure

Sohan Singh Hayreh, Wayne March, Douglas R. Anderson

University of Iowa, Department of Ophthalmology, Iowa City, Iowa 52242, USA

Although axoplasmic flow blockage (AFB) with raised intraocular pressure (IOP) is well-established (1-11), its pathogenesis remains an enigma. AFB may be due to ischemia of the optic nerve fibers (6) or mechanical axonal compression (8). The present study was designed to determine whether the AFB is due to ischemia or mechanical compression of the optic nerve fibers in the optic nerve head.

Materials and Methods

In 40 young adult healthy rhesus monkeys, the perfusion pressure (PP) in the eyes was altered by several methods:

a) Perfusion pump method: in 32 animals a pump with adjustable speed was used to perfuse blood from the descending aorta into the right common carotid artery to manipulate (usually to elevate) the blood pressure (BP) in the right eye. The following cannulations were done in these animals:

1) A cannula was introduced via one femoral artery into the upper part of the descending aorta and connected to a pressure transducer to measure the systemic BP.

2) A cannula introduced via the other femoral artery into the upper part of the descending aorta was connected via a tube passing through the perfusion pump to the right common carotid artery.

3) The right common carotid artery was ligated in the neck; a cannula was introduced in the upper cranial part of the artery and tied in position. This cannula was connected by a T tube to the tube from the perfusion pump and to a transducer to measure the BP.

4) The left common carotid artery was cannulated by a T tube, which allowed measurement of the PB with a transducer without blocking the flow of the blood from the heart to the cranial cavacity.

5) A cannula was introduced through the right femoral vein into the upper part of the inferior vena cava and was used to administer additional anesthetic, heparin, etc.

6) The anterior chamber of each eye was cannulated by a 30-gauge needle via a cannula was connected separately to a reservoir and a transducer. The pressure transducers were connected to an eight-channel Beckman RM Dynograph Recorder for a continuous recording of the various pressures.

b) Production of systemic arterial hypotension by giving intravenously ganglion-blocking drugs: this was successful in two of seven animals where it was attempted.

c) Production of systemic arterial hypotension by bleeding: this was attempted in some animals and succeeded in only one animal.

d) Production of systemic arterial hypertension: this was attempted by administration of angiotensin and allied compounds but could not be adequately maintained for the duration of the experiment.

The animals were fully heparinized. Two types of studies were performed in all:

1) Fluorescein angiographic studies on the optic disk and posterior fundus were performed within 5 min after elevating the IOP to a desired height in each eye, first in one eye and then in the other. A few days before this experiment, all eyes had normal angiographic studies performed to serve as a baseline for comparison.

2) Axoplasmic flow blockage studies were performed shortly after the angiographic studies; 0.1 ml (100 μCi) of tritiated leucine was injected into the vitreous in front of the macular region in both eyes of all animals by the method described by ANDERSON and HENDRICKSON (1). The IOPs and the BP in the right common carotid artery were adjusted to the desired level. The animal was perfused with buffered glutaraldehyde fixative through the carotid cannulae 6 - 7.5h after the injection of the tritiated leucine (or earlier in some animals that did not survive the entire desired length of the experiment). The eyes were enucleated and sent from Iowa City to Miami for light microscopic autoradiographic studies by the technique described by ANDERSON and HENDRICKSON (1). The investigator at Miami evaluated the degree of block of axonal transport without knowing the experimental condition of the particular eye.

Observations and Discussion

To answer the question of whether AFB is a direct mechanical effect or is mediated by ischemia, the basis for analyzing the data is to determine whether the presence of AFB (and the degree of AFB) relates more closely to the level of IOP (which would suggest a mechanical basis) or to PP (which would suggest an ischemic mechanism). Several biologic and technical variables confound the data interpretation. These must be kept in mind and need to be reviewed before considering the meaning of the data itself.

First, PP calculated from the carotid artery BP differs somewhat from the PP in the vascular system in the optic nerve head (due to distance along the vascular pathway, anatomic variability in blood supply to the nerve head, and variability in intracranial anastomotic connections, for example in the circle of Willis). Furthermore, there may be a variable relationship between PP and nutritive blood flow, depending on the age, physiologic state of the animal, and drug effects in the anesthetized animals. The blood flow and the nutritive capability of a given PP may vary from one range of BP to another; for example, a PP of 35 mm Hg due to a BP of 110 mm Hg and an IOP of 75 mm Hg may not be the same as that due to a BP of 50 mm Hg and an IOP of 15 mm Hg. Similarly, no definite information is available about the effect on the axoplasmic flow of lowering the PP from a normal level (about 85 mm Hg) down to various levels. During a 6-h experiment, it was almost impossible to maintain a constant BP.

Secondly, the use of a perfusion pump in the right carotid system may do more than affect the BP and pulse rate on the right side, although we had not anticipated this possibility when designing the experiment. The pump may cause a release of vasoactive substances such as serotonin (Bill, personal communication), promote formation of thrombi, or have undesirable tissue effects due to overperfusion or very fast rate combined with an abnormally high pulse pressure. These may be counterproductive to the nourishment or function of axons on the right side despite a higher BP.

Finally, it must be kept in mind that there are important limitations in quantifying AFB because of biologic variations (producing different grades of AFB in different bundles that are randomly selected in a single histologic slide or two that was examined), lack of accurate assessment of AFB, and observer variability in grading the degree of AFB. These limitations of this study and the lack of an absolute correlation between AFB and PP or IOP in this study introduce many ambiguities; the results could be interpreted several ways, depending upon one's bias.

Of more than 40 animals subjected to the experiments, 13 were technically unsatisfactory. These had labile blood pressures, died too early in the experiment, or were otherwise unsuitable. It is convenient to consider the remaining 27 animals in two groups:

Group I: in 19 monkeys, the IOP was maintained at the same level in the two eyes. In all animals but one, blood was perfused into the right common carotid artery by the perfusion pump. The rate of the pump pulsation was $2\frac{1}{2}$ to 3 times that of the normal heart rate. The systolic BP was usually higher and the diastolic BP lower on the side of the pump as compared to the left common carotid artery and systemic BP.

Group II: in eight monkeys, the IOP was not equal in the two eyes. In one animal, the perfusion pump had been used. Another monkey developed systemic arterial hypotension following massive blood loss at the start of the experiment. The remaining six monkeys had been given hexamethonium or an allied drug in an attempt to produce systemic arterial hypotension, though this was achieved successfully only in two of the animals. The PP in the two eyes was maintained at different levels by altering the IOPs.

Generally, it seems that AFB did not occur if the IOP was less than 30 mm Hg, even if the PP was very low by virtue of a very low BP. However, seven eyes of four animals were exceptions, showing definite AFB with IOPs of 5, 14, 14, 15, 15, 21, and 30 mm Hg, and in these the AFB can be attributed to a low PP. Furthermore, there were five eyes of five animals that failed to show definite AFB with high IOP (36, 40, 45, 60, and 68 mm Hg). From these exceptions at both ends of the IOP scale, it is evident that there is an imperfect relationship between IOP and the occurrence of AFB. This would be further suggested by four animals of Group I with no AFB in one eye but a definite AFB in the fellow eye, in spite of the equally elevated IOP in the two eyes, (30, 36, 45, and 68 mm Hg); the eye with the AFB had a lower PP in all of them.

On the other hand, there is also an imperfect correlation between AFB and PP. At one end of the scale, several eyes failed to show a block with low PP (between 10 and 40 mm Hg) unless the IOP was greater than 30 mm Hg, suggesting that there may be a possible combination of factors entering into the manifestation of AFB. At the other end of the scale were six eyes of five animals with good PP (over 55 mm Hg) and high IOP (over 45 mm Hg), showing AFB that would be attributed to high IOP. Of note, however, is that five of these six were right eyes, being perfused with the pump, and we cannot be sure whether AFB in these eyes occurred due to a high IOP or to the above-mentioned effects of the pump. This separation could be made only in left eyes (without a pump) with good PP and a high IOP. In such eyes, AFB could be attributed to high IOP and the lack of AFB to the absence of the pump, but no such eyes were in this experimental series.

Overall, in a scatterplot of eyes without a pump (left eyes of Group I and all but one eye of Group II), the degree of AFB related loosely with both a high IOP and a low PP, as had been true in a previous series (1). It cannot be determined whether AFB related better to PP or IOP because IOP and PP correlate inversely with one another over the narrow range of spontaneously occurring BP. The effects of IOP and PP could be separated only by successfully manipulating BP, as was attempted in the eyes with the pump in this study. Unfortunately, the pump created its own artifacts.

In two animals of group II with equal PP in the two eyes of each animal, the AFB was more marked in the eye with lower IOP in one animal, the reverse in the second animal.

In group I, where both eyes had equal IOP, the PP was the only variable between the two eyes. In this group an attempt might be made to study whether the eye with more marked AFB had lower PP or showed no such pattern. The results of such an analysis are shown in Table 1. More marked AFB associated with lower PP was seen in ten animals (on left side in eight and right side in two). In four animals, the more marked AFB was in the eye with higher PP and in all of them this occurred in the right eye and could be blamed on the artifacts (hence ischemia) produced by the pump. In Table 1 all exceptions to the expected pattern (i.e., more marked AFB in the eye with lower PP) are in the direction of favoring a greater

Table 1. Correlation[a] between the eye with more marked AFB and lower PP among the two eyes of 19 monkeys of group I, with equal IOP in the two eyes

	Eye with (in number of animals)		
Lower PP	More marked axoplasmic flow block		
	Right eye	Equally marked	Left eye
Right eye	2	None	None
Equally marked	None	2	None
Left eye	4	3	8

[a] P = 0.0898[13]

AFB in the right eye, and none are in the inverse direction. Noteworthy is that among the eight animals with a greater block on the left, all had a lower PP on the left. This could be argued as a chance happening since in fact nearly all (15 of 17) animals with unequal PP had a lower PP on the left. Nonetheless, both animals with a lower PP on the right had greater AFB on the right, and while two animals is too few to rely on, this finding, together with the greater AFB in eight animals in the left eye with lower PP, is somewhat suggestive of an ischemic basis for AFB. On statistical analysis (12), there is a suggestive relationship between AFB and PP in Table 1, although the probability value (P = 0.09) fails to reach the accepted level of statistical significance. It could be argued that availability of accurate techniques of estimation of AFB and PP in the optic nerve head and elimination of probable artifacts introduced by the perfusion pump might have "improved" the positive correlation.

Some eyes showed variations and inconsistencies that favored neither the ischemic nor the mechanical theories. These may represent biologic variations that did not follow the mathematic expectations, or may be examples of the variability of the methods of detecting and quantifying AFB, or there may be some other unknown factor(s) operating.

It may be pertinent to refer very briefly to the relevant findings of fluorescein fundus angiographic studies in these animals. These revealed delay in the filling of the choroidal vascular bed on altering the PP and the delay showed a significant relationship with PP ($P = 0.002$) but not with IOP ($P = 0.537$). Since the blood supply to the prelaminar part of the optic nerve head usually comes from the peripapillary choroid, the data was further analyzed for the circulatory delay in the various parts of the peripapillary choroid. This showed that eyes with peripapillary choroidal delay had about half the PP of those showing no such delay (45 ± 16 mm Hg), but the mean IOP in both the groups was about equal (about 50 mm Hg). This is further suggestive of ischemic mechanism.

In summary, this study has been inconclusive in resolving the controversy between the ischemic and mechanical theories. Raising BP in the right common carotid artery with the perfusion pump failed to protect the right eye in a majority of the animals from AFB produced by elevated IOP. We do not know whether this means that AFB is not dependent upon PP or whether the beneficial effect of a higher BP was negated by an adverse effect of the pump on the perfused optic nerve head. Although no single observation is absolutely decisive one way or the other, the sum total of the various evidence put together is somewhat suggestive that the AFB in the present study was probably mediated by ischemic mechanism, e.g., occurrence of AFB in several animals with low PP without elevated IOP, absence of AFB in some eyes with high IOP, and fluorescein angiographic evidence of peripapillary choroidal delay related to PP but not to IOP, etc. The possibility of some other factor(s) operating cannot be excluded completely. This study in no way enters into the controversy of whether AFB has any role to play in the optic nerve head changes in glaucoma.

Acknowledgements

This investigation was supported in part by Public Health Service research grant EY-01576 (Dr. Hayreh) and EY-00031 (Dr. Anderson) awarded by the National Eye Institute, Bethesda, Maryland. Dr. Anderson is a Research to Prevent Blindness-William and Mary Greve Scholar. We are grateful to Mr. James Swaner for the technical assistance and to Miss Jane Duwa for the secretarial assistance.

References

(1) Anderson, D.R.; Hendrickson, A.: Effect of intraocular pressure on rapid axoplasmic transport in monkey optic nerve. Invest. Ophthalmol. 13, 771-783 (1974)

(2) Anderson, D.R.; Hendrickson, A.E.: Failure of increased intracranial pressure to affect rapid axonal transport at the optic nerve head. Invest. Ophthalmol. Vis. Sci. 16, 423-426 (1977)

(3) Hansson, H.A.: Glial reactions induced by treatment with colchicine of central nervous system of rabbits. Acta Neuropathol. (Berl.) 22, 145-157 (1972)

(4) Hansson, H.A.: Uptake and intracellular bidirectional transport of horseradish peroxidase in retinal ganglion cells. Exp. Eye. Res. 16, 377-388 (1973)

(5) Lampert, P.W.; Vogel, M.H.; Zimmermann, L.E.: Pathology of the optic nerve in experimental acute glaucoma: Electron microscopic studies. Invest. Ophthalmol. 7, 199-213 (1968)

(6) Levy, N.S.: Functional implications of axoplasmic transport. Invest. Ophthalmol. 13, 639-640 (1974)

(7) Levy, N.S.: The effects of elevated intraocular pressure on slow axonal protein flow. Invest. Ophthalmol. 13, 691-695 (1976)

(8) Minckler, D.S.; Bunt, A.H.; Johanson, G.W.: Orthograde and retrograde axoplasmic transport during acute ocular hypertension in the monkey. Invest. Ophthalmol. Vis. Sci. 16, 426-441 (1977)

(9) Minckler, D.S.; Tso, M.O.M.; Zimmerman, L.E.: A light microscopic, autoradiographic study of axoplasmic transport in the optic nerve head during ocular hypotony, increased intraocular pressure and papilledema. Am. J. Ophthalmol. 82, 741-757 (1976)

(10) Quigley, H.A.; Anderson, D.R.: The dynamics and location of axonal transport blockade by acute intraocular pressure elevation in primate optic nerve. Invest. Ophthalmol. 15, 606-616 (1976)

(11) Quigley, H.A.; Anderson, D.R.: Distribution of axonal transport blockade by acute intraocular pressure elevation in the primate optic nerve head. Invest. Ophthal. Vis. Sci. 16, 640-644 (1977)

(12) Conover, W.J.: Practical nonparametric statistics. p. 368, Table III. New York: Wiley 1971

Discussion

LEYDHECKER: I should like to congratulate Dr. HAYREH on his honesty in demonstrating and critically discussing an enormous work with no conclusive results. This might prevent a further loss of grey hair for future investigators and a loss of dollars to the public.

BRUBAKER: It is possible to control the blood pressure in the head of the rhesus monkey in the following way. A pressure cuff is placed around both common carotid arteries in the neck. A distal artery, such as the facial, is used to monitor pressure in the head of the animal. A servocontrol system is used to inflate the cuffs to the pressure necessary to maintain the arterial blood pressure in the sentinal vessel at a predetermined level (below the undisturbed arterial pressure). The intraocular pressure can be controlled independently in each eye by two other servocontrol systems. Thus, intraocular pressure and perfusion pressure can be controlled independently in this animal without pumping blood or using systemically administered pharmacologic agents.

HAYREH: Monkeys have an arterial trunk that connects the two ophthalmic arteries intracranially so that altering the blood pressure in the common carotid artery may not necessarily alter the perfusion pressure in the optic nerve head.

ERNEST: We know that to inhibit nerve conduction by direct pressure on the nerve itself requires several hundred mm Hg far outside the physiologic range. What is known of the functional significance of the blockage of axoplasmic flow?

HAYREH: I did not want to enter into the controversy of the role of axoplasmic flow block in optic disk-cupping and visual loss. My personal view is that the available evidence show that axoplasmic flow block has no role to play in the optic disk changes, as discussed in my previous publications. We know that axoplasmic flow has no role to play in the conduction of the impulse along an axon because the impulse travels along the membrane of the axon and not along the axoplasm. Moreover, all the available evidence clearly shows that axoplasmic flow block, even for months or years, does not produce any functional loss, e.g., in optic disk edema due to raised intracranial pressure; experimental studies also support this.

BILL: We have gathered some experience in cynomolgus monkeys that may be of interest in this context. When we tried to produce a difference in carotid arterial blood pressure by ligating one carotid, we found that this was rather ineffective. We then tried to withdraw blood from the distal part of the divided carotid artery hoping to obtain a marked difference in ophthalmic arterial pressure. But even then the difference produced was small. It seems, therefore, that the arterial anastomoses in the circle of Willis and possibly elsewhere tend to equalize the ophthalmic arterial pressures. To produce marked differences, one will probably have to ligate these anastomoses in addition to the interference with the carotid artery.

HAYREH: I would confirm Dr. BILL's observations. This has a clinical application in patients with carotid artery disease; I have been frequently asked about how I explain the lack of optic disk changes in such patients if the optic disk-cupping is due to vascular insufficiency. Our observations clearly show that occlusion or narrowing of the carotid artery is not always accompanied by poor perfusion in the optic disk.

LANGHAM: We have been investigating the same questions, i.e., the effect of perfusion pressure on visual function. We have investigated more than 70 patients with significant stenosis of one or both carotid arteries. We have measured the intraocular pressure and the opthalmic pressure and have found the ocular perfusion pressures (ophthalmic systolic pressure-intraocular pressure) to range 10 - 40 mm Hg depending on the severity of the disease. This compares with the mean ocular perfusion pressure of 75 mm Hg in normal patients and values of 60 - 80 mm Hg found in a group of open-angle glaucoma patients with field loss and cupping of the disk. In patients with carotid occlusive disease, there was no glaucomatous disk-cupping or field loss even in those patients who had minimal perfusion pressure for periods exceeding 1 year.

HAYREH: The patients with arterial hypertension belong to a totally different group as compared to those with carotid artery disease, and the two should not be mixed. As regards the carotid artery disease and lack of optic disk-cupping, no doubt one comes across patients where in carotid artery occlusion, particularly in bilateral carotid artery disease, there is optic disk-cupping. The absence of cupping in these patients is not at all surprising because if the occlusive process is slow (and unilateral), collateral channels open up intracranially to compensate for the carotid artery occlusion or stenosis. In eyes with lower than normal perfusion pressure, in these patients, as indicated by Dr. LANGHAM, the absence of optic disk-cupping may be due to lack of ischemia, and the lower perfusion pressure may be enough to maintain good nutrition; a fall of perfusion pressure to a certain extent may not always produce damage. We need a large, unbiased, randomly selected sample to get accurate information.

We tried to produce systemic arterial hypotension in monkeys by various methods, none of which proved successful. The majority of rhesus monkey do not respond to ganglion-blocking agents because in only two of about a dozen was some fall in blood pressure with ganglion-blocking agents observed; this was totally an unexpected finding. We tried to produce the hypotension by bleeding the animal, and most of these animals died of shock and were of no use in this study. We tried to produce arterial hypertension by drugs, but the effect of the drugs lasted less than 1 h and the drugs had no effect whatsoever after that. Thus, there are tremendous amounts of technical limitations in conducting such an experiment.

Summary Report of "Biostatistical Analysis of the Collaborative Glaucoma Study"

Mansour F. Armaly, Dean Krueger, Cindy Maunder

George Washington University, Medical Center, Dept. of Ophthalmology
2150 Pennsyvania Ave., Washington, D.C. 20037, USA

Each of you should have received by mail a copy of the final report entitled, "Biostatistical Analysis of the Collaborative Glaucoma Study". I hope you have had a chance to study this voluminous and detailed report so that only a brief summary will be needed at this time. The Collaborative Glaucoma Study, included the following investigators and centers during the period 1959 - 1973:

Mansour F. Armaly, M.D., University of Iowa, Iowa City, Iowa
Bernard Becker, M.D., Washington University, St. Louis, Missouri
Ralph Levine, M.D., New York University, New York, New York
Irvin Pollack, M.D., Johns Hopkins University, Baltimore, Maryland
Robert Schaeffer, M .D., University of California, San Francisco

During this period, the Collaborative Study was supported in part by various grants and contracts from the Bureau of State Services, National Institute of Neurological Disease and Blindness, and the National Eye Institute.

The objective of this study was to investigate the value of various tests of ocular fluid dynamics and certain ocular traits in predicting the future development of glaucomatous visual field defects. A fixed protocol describing the criteria of recruitment of appropriate subjects as well as the details of each test and the standardization of the sequence of performance of these tests as well as their interpretation was developed jointly by the principal investigators.

Participating subjects were free from visual field defects or abnormalities that could interfere with the validity of any of the tests. The majority of them were relatives of known glaucoma patients because of the expectation that the incidence of field defects in the future will be higher in them than in the general population; the group also included subjects known to have elevated intraocular pressure but free from field defects as well as subjects recruited from the general population.

Yearly standardized examination was performed on these subjects until the development of a defined field defect. Since no prior experience with suitable methods for epidemiologic studies of glaucoma in a large population was present at that time, the development of the protocol was a gradual one and involved first the tests that were best known and last the ones that were in the process of standardization. To this last group belonged the examination of the visual field. The last change in this test was a major one and went into effect at the beginning of 1968 and involved the collection of standardized records and the analysis of the records themselves rather than the descriptive terms of the individual physician.

As different parts of the protocol became standardized, the standardized tests were taught to each technician in the participating centers and their performance supervised regularly and frequently to insure the continued adherence to the standardized procedure in a uniform fashion among the different centers. All data were centrally collected for computer analysis. The batter of tests included a detailed as well as a brief medical and ocular history, examination of the visual acuity with and without correction, general physical examination of both eyes, specifically, including specific observations on the cornea, anterior chamber, iris, lens, vitreous, retina, and optic disk and recording applanation tonometry, tonography before water-drinking test as well as after water-drinking test, and finally, standardized perimetry.

About 6000 subjects were entered into the study, and their records were reviewed in detail by the analytic staff for possible errors, inconsistencies, and the like, as well as for the actual coding and description of the visual field from the original record. A series of 12 types of visual field abnormalities were identified, objective criteria for identification of each type were developed, and all Goldmann perimeter charts for a selected sample of about 1000 subjects were reviewed; these facts were coded in accordance with the objective criteria. This review produced a set of data on visual field defects that were useful in developing alternative definitions of glaucomatous visual field defects for analytic purposes. These definitions were subsequently tested for association with potential risk factors for glaucoma. They included the following: (1) nasal step of more than 10° in the peripheral or in the central visual field; (2) scotoma to the threshold slip stimulus with depth of I/3e on the Goldmann perimeter or more and one step or more above the threshold stimulus (a step means a difference of 0.5 log unit); (3) blind spot enlargement of more than 90° to the threshold stimulus or the I/2e with depth of more than I/3e and more than one step above threshold stimulus.

Ninety-eight eyes were found to have developed one or more of the above defects during their participation in the study. These eyes were used together with the total sample to identify characteristics of study subjects and eyes as measured at the beginning of the study that are associated with the subsequent occurrence of glaucomatous field defect by means of univarient logistic function coefficients. Applanation pressure, outflow facility, change in pressure after water-drinking test, cup/disk ratio, and age were identified as the major associated variables excluding some that either measured the same phenomenon (such as applanation pressure and Schiotz pressure) or are highly correlated (such as age and the presence of lens opacity). Incidence rates of glaucomatous field defect at each of several levels of each variable were calculated and showed strong consistent gradients of increase in incidence with increase in initial value of applanation pressure, reduction in outflow facility, increase in pressure rise after water drinking, increase in cup/disk ratio, and older age. Incidence rates for combinations of levels of each pair of risk factors showed strong joint effects but often weaker effects of one factor at a high level of the other.

Rates of incidence of each of the defects comprising glaucomatous visual field types and of each of eight other types of visual field abnormalities in relation to levels of applanation pressure, outflow facility, and age were calculated and led to a decision to neither contract or expand the definition of glaucomatous visual field defects. This decision was reinforced by comparison for each of the types of visual field abnormalities of the mean values of each of the risk factors for eyes with and for eyes without the abnormality.

The multiple logistic risk function is a device for multivariate analysis of data in which the dependent or outcome variable is dichotomous, in this instance, the occurrence or nonoccurrence of glaucomatous field defect. This method was used to derive coefficients that estimate the influence of each of a set of factors on an outcome when the set of factors are considered together. Each of the five factors make an important separate contribution to risk the order of size of risk being age, followed by outflow facility, followed by applanation pressure, followed by cup/disk ratio and finally, by pressure rise after the water-drinking test. The coefficient for age is about five times the coefficient for pressure rise after the water-drinking test. Introduction of each of several other factors as fixed variables had little effect on results and led to the conclusion that predictive power would not be substantially improved if more of the studied variables were included in the analysis.

While risk factors were analyzed separately for each clinic, there was no statistically significant difference amongst clinic and, therefore, the data of all clinics were pooled together for statistical analysis. Values of risk factors were calculated separately for eyes with transient defects and eyes with untransient defects. For transient defects, age and applanation pressure were clearly the dominant risk factors.

All risk factor analyses were based on the average value of risk factors at the first and second examination for both defect and nondefect eyes. There was an average interval of 6.5 years for the first examination to first occurrence of defect in the 98 eyes. To determine whether risk factor relationships changed as the time interval to defect shortened, we identified a subset of eyes for which there was a minimum of 5 years from first examination to examination at which a defect first occurred. Multivarient coefficients based on values of the five risk factors recorded 5 years, 3 years, and 1 year prior to the defect on last examination showed only modest changes. Thus, there is no evidence from this study that occurrence of glaucomatous visual field defects as defined in this analysis is heralded by marked changes in applanation pressure, outflow facility, or pressure rise after water-drinking test or the cup/disk ratio.

The multivarient coefficients can be applied to the values of the risk factors recorded for individual eyes to produce a calculated probability of occurrence of glaucomatous visual field defect in each eye. When this is done, the majority of eyes has small calculated probabilities (less than 0.02), which is consistent with an overall incidence of glaucomatous defect of 1.7% during the course of the study. Only 13% of the eyes that did develop glaucomatous field defect have calculated probabilities of 0.10 or greater. Nevertheless, the distribution of eyes with field defects and those without are markedly different indicating that the five risk factors have important predictive power even though it is clear that other factors that influence the occurrence of glaucomatous visual field defects were not recorded in this study. The probability distribution of eyes for which only transient defects were recorded was more like the distribution of eyes that were not associated with glaucomatous field defect than that of eyes with nontransient glaucomatous visual field defects.

Life table techniques were used to calculate the proportions of eyes that remained free of glaucomatous visual field defect for successive numbers of years of observation, for groups of eyes classified according to initial values of applanation pressure and of outflow facility.

Conclusion

The data recorded in this study are considered adequate to identify five important risk factors for glaucomatous visual field defects and to conclude that a substantial number of other variables are not sufficiently important to warrant further investigation. The ability of the five factors to predict the particular eyes in which glaucomatous field defects would occur is disappointingly low. Large proportions of glaucomatous visual field defects occurred in eyes for which the values of individual risk factor: applanation pressure, outflow facility, change in pressure after water-drinking test, and cup/disk ratio were "normal." The levels of risk factors rather than their change with time during the observation in this study appear to be the important element of its contribution to risk. Characteristics, ocular and otherwise, that were not recorded in the study undoubtedly affect the occurrence of glaucoma.

KRIEGLSTEIN: To me the most important point to be derived from follow-up studies is the relationship between intraocular pressure and the probability of field loss. If there is a linear relationship, it would be difficult to use intraocular pressure as an indicator for therapy. However, provided there is a nonlinear relationship, the pressure range where the curve bends over would be decisive for therapy (Fig.1).

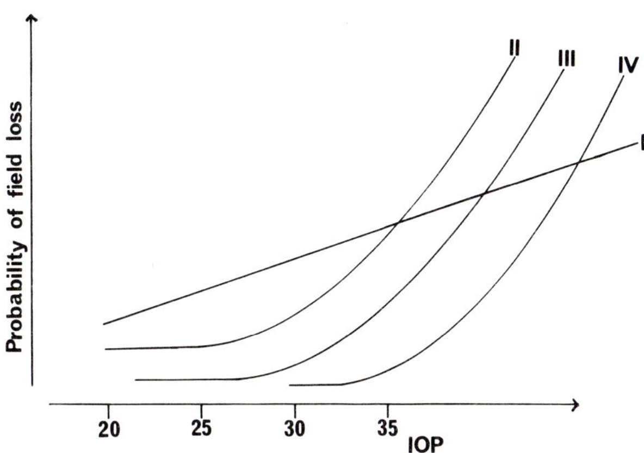

Fig.1. Hypothetical possible relationships between intraocular pressure and the probability of visual field loss. I indicates a linear relationship, II, III, and IV a nonlinear relationship. The bendover point of the curve would correspond to the individual tension tolerance limit.

Discussion

BENGTSSON: As to the question on what could be done differently in another prospective study I have to confess that I am already in the process of performing one. My answer would be: an unselected population of subjects 55 - 70 years old should be surveyed by a single investigator. Automatic perimetry and fundus photography are indispensable. The goal has to be early detection rather than prediction.

KITAZAWA: You stated that 45% of your cases who later developed field defects had an intraocular pressure of less than 20 mm Hg at first. On the basis of your results, do you think that intraocular pressure is not useful in predicting the outcome in each individual? If so, what do you think is the most reliable factor for the prediction of prognosis in each case?

LEYDHECKER: I wish to congratulate Dr. ARMALY on the enormous amount of work that he has invested in his study. Even if the results are not as clear-cut as we wished, still just this result is important enough. I have two questions: 1) Was the interobserver variation of perimetrists tested? 2) Can we conclude from your study that a pressure of 20 mm Hg should ring a bell in our head, that we should do a visual field examination and ask the patient to come back for a follow-up? Or can we tell him that he is still within normal limits of pressure and needs no further special examination such as a visual field study?
There is one parameter that differentiates two kinds of response in eyes with pressures between 18 and 22 mm Hg. This is my tonographic test lasting 7 min. I agree that the value of C or P/C for 4 min tonography is not of much use for separating such eyes into two different groups. The reason is that during the first 3 min of tonography too many different reactions occur that have not much to do with glaucoma, e.g., the suppression of secretion by the pressure increase and shifting of the blood from the eye. However, during the last 4 min of the 7-min tonography, these reactions have calmed down and the eye has found a new equilibrium. I use this tonographic test to differentiate between normal and abnormal reactions. However, I am not able to tell whether these reactions are predictors as regards the loss of visual field, but it might be wise to include a 7-min tonography instead of 4-min study in future research.

KITAZAWA: I presume that you came to select five predictors on the basis of discriminating efficiency of each predictor. As a result, I believe you have a discriminant function for prediction. Now there are several prospective studies available, and I wonder if you have used the data of those prospective studies to evaluate the validity of your discriminant function.

HAYREH: What would you consider a safe intraocular pressure when you can say the patient does not need a careful follow-up in the future? So far, most of us have done that with intraocular pressures of about 20 mm Hg.

ZIMMERMAN: Looking back, what would you do differently in design, methods, goal, etc.?

MISHIMA: Statistical studies on large numbers of cases are of extreme importance in many respects, one of which may be the understanding of the evolution of the disease and prediction of its process. When we see patients at the first visit, we do not know the previous history of the particular patients. For this reason and also for evolution of treatment, it is of interest to analyze the evolution by calender years. How do you indicate the years in your graph in calculation of the probability of the field loss and its yearly increase?

AULHORN: 1) I am very impressed by the enormous amount of data in your study, but I think the significance of the relationship between visual field defects and all the other factors depends on the quality of your perimetry. Are the perimetrists trained in the same way? In which way are they trained?
2) I think the term "nasal step" should be better defined. What you call "nasal step." I would define as a scotoma in the nasal field. There are then really no differences in our findings of the location of the earliest field defects.

SHAFFER: In clinical practice, it would not be feasible to perform complete visual field studies on all patients with a pressure of 20 mm Hg. One's whole time would be spent doing fields. Only if other suspicious signs were present would I consider such a patient to be at high risk.

ARMALY: Dr. MISHIMA's question: The answer is that year in study not calender year was used in the life table analysis.
Dr. DRANCE's question: The five predictors are indeed poor predictors. However, they are predictors nevertheless. They are the best of the 26 factors we looked at, yet they do not predict a majority of the eyes likely to develop field loss. It is important to point out that as we attempt to identify other predictors in the future we should avoid wasting any effort in studying factors that have a high correlation with any of the five variables of our study. That is why I will not be enthusiastic about drug effects that correlate with pressure level.
Dr. AULHORN's comment is obviously crucial. Since the end point of the study is a visual field defect, the methods of perimetry become the corner stone of validity of the study. There is no question that now we can design a better method than we did

in 1959 and the mid-1960s. However, we used the method described in the protocol, and all technicians in the different centers were first trained in the method, then evaluated for performance. Study sessions and evaluation sessions involving all technicians were conducted at regular intervals several times a year to insure continued high quality of performance. The question of nasal step or scotoma is simply answered by referring you to the definition in the protocol. A scotoma is a defect within the isopter, a nasal step is a configuration of the isopter boundary. A nasal step for one isopter or test object may be scotoma within a larger isopter.
In answer to Dr. LEYDHECKER, it is true that 20 mm Hg or greater should ring a bell. The question is what will the bell tell me. It tells me the patient should have a careful visual field and description of optic disk. If these are found normal, then I recommend to them that they have repeated evaluation every 6 - 8 months because they have a higher possibility of developing field loss in the future. This is especially true if other risk factors are also present, such as family history of glaucoma, large cup, myopia, etc. The ringing bell does not mean to begin some sort of drug therapy.
Dr. KITAZAWA's question must be answered in the negative. Unfortunately, we did not have the opportunity to apply or test our discriminant function to a completely new study. We did the internal check we reported in the distributed report, and it showed good agreement.
Dr. KRIEGLSTEIN's question about the increase in incidence for higher pressure level: There is greater increase in frequency after 27 mm Hg. But remember that the vast majority of cases are already below 27 mm Hg even though the percent incidence may be greater. We should always think of number of cases rather than percent.
Dr. BILL's question: We have a general listing of drugs used but did not include it in the analysis; specifically alcohol was not looked for.
Looking back, in response to Dr. ZIMMERMANN, the design of the study will be tighter, the methodology more standardized, and whenever possible subjective judgment replaced by objective recording. Dr. BENGTSSON has already described some of the improvements in his study.

Present Trends in Glaucoma Research

Steven M. Podos

Mount Sinai School of Medicine, Department of Ophthalmology, New York City, N.Y., USA

The major discoveries pertaining to a disease process are firmly rooted in a scientific milieu of basic observations, often from diverse and apparently unrelated sources (5). Thus, being asked to review results in recent glaucoma research that are of greatest importance and on which areas such investigations should concentrate in the future may produce answers that are both presumptuous and misleading. Nevertheless, one can try to point out major problems, give examples of progress made in areas stressing basic and clinical interactions, and in so doing suggest many more questions that need to be answered. In brief summary fashion, necessarily incomplete, I shall attempt to do this for the disease primary open-angle glaucoma, considering etiology and pathogenesis, diagnosis and therapy.

The cause of primary open-angle glaucoma is unknown. The etiology of the glaucomatous process may relate to many factors (11), or we may be dealing with a family of diseases. One obvious common theme is an elevation of intraocular pressure. Why does this occur? What is the site of the defect? The trabecular meshwork and Schlemm's canal appear to be the most likely areas. Some suggest a mechanical hypothesis, invoking defects in the vacuolar process or a peculiar collapsability of these structures (14, 20). Others mention biochemical abnormalities. However, at present there is no evidence that the outflow channels in open-angle glaucomatous eyes differ biochemically or histopathologically from eyes of older individuals without glaucoma. Many areas need further examination in this regard. The relationship of hypersensitivity to corticosteroids and primary open-angle glaucoma is of continuing interest. The increased intraocular pressure response induced by corticosteroids in eyes with open-angle glaucoma (2) and the suggested hypersensitivity to corticosteroids of lymphocytes from patients with primary open-angle glaucoma (4) may be clues to the elucidation of the disease. Also, what is the role of mucopolysaccharides (7), can we identify differences in various enzymes in the abnormal trabecular structure, and are there ultrastructural or functional alterations involving microfilaments or microtubules in glaucomatous tissue or tissue from corticosteroid-sensitive eyes?

The notion that the ocular damage in open-angle glaucoma depends upon an imbalance of intraocular pressure and blood supply to the optic nerve shifts the emphasis from intraocular pressure to the anatomic and physiologic status of the optic nerve. A given level of intraocular pressure may lead to functional loss in one individual but not in another or in the same individual at one but not another time. Optic nerve destruction in primary open-angle glaucoma may be a result of vascular insufficiency (13). Fluorescein angiograms done at different intraocular pressure levels in a given eye suggest that the choroidal circulation is particularly susceptible to increased intraocular pressure in glaucoma. Unfortunately, the variability inherent in fluorescein angiography limits its usefulness in demonstrating early vascular insufficiency of the optic nerve head circulation. On the other hand, mechanical factors may be primarily responsible for optic nerve damage. For instance, obstruction of axoplasmic transport in the region of the lamina cribosa is induced by moderate elevation of intraocular pressure (1). Although these observations do not indicate whether the pathogenesis of the damage is vascular or mechanical, they are worth further study. An imbalance between intraocular pressure and cerebrospinal fluid pressure may be responsible for such a mechanical alteration in the optic nerve (YABLONSKI and KRUPIN, unpublished).

The crucial diagnostic problem involves the decision to initiate therapy for primary open-angle glaucoma. The loss of visual function in open-angle glaucoma may not depend upon the intraocular pressure level alone but also upon other modifying factors. Some of these factors are extraocular and involve vascular, metabolic, endocrine, and genetic considerations. Many of the known factors are ocular. Documentation of these presents other problems. Our future understanding of the problem of primary open-angle glaucoma will depend upon our ability to identify the relevant factors and the mechanism by which they influence the onset and course of the disease process.

Much of the philosophy of withholding therapy in patients with no visible or documentable damage is based on the results of prospective studies of patients with intraocular pressures in the 20s and 30s followed for up to 10 years. Additional and longer prospective studies are needed to increase our ability to predict which individuals with ocular hypertension will develop glaucomatous damage. In general, the higher the intraocular pressure and the longer it is present, the greater the chance for damage to occur. However, while elevated intraocular pressure is an extremely important factor in the natural history of primary open-angle glaucoma, there is no simple relationship between the intraocular pressure level and the development of subsequent ocular damage. Diagnostic tests are being sought to identify which eyes at what pressure levels are susceptible, such as the sophisticated fluorescein analyses of GOLDMANN (10). Such techniques also would allow investigation of methods to increase the resistance of the optic nerve head to pressure damage. Another suggestion involves the possible prognostic significance of a pressure response to epinephrine (3). The results of such methods may drastically alter our ability to detect and treat primary open-angle glaucoma.

One argument against withholding therapy in the glaucoma suspect is the possibility that an eye once damaged is less resistant to further damage from elevated intraocular pressure. A recent small study suggests that an eye with an established field defect may be more susceptible at a given intraocular pressure level to further damage than an eye at the same intraocular pressure level without field loss (12).

Finally, one must raise the issue of whether or not reduction of intraocular pressure prevents the development or progression of glaucomatous visual field defects. Until we know the cause of primary open-angle glaucoma, we will have difficulty preventing and treating its manifestations.

The identification of the early field defects in primary open-angle glaucoma, of utmost importance for rational management, is not satisfactory. Static perimetry is an accurate method of determining threshold sensitivity in selected meridians. Automated perimetry is another current investigative tool (6). The ideal method for visual field testing, an objective, rapid, and inexpensive device, is yet to be developed. Similarly, we are hampered by inadequate delineation of the optic nerve head. Experimental photogrammetric means of depicting the optic cup offer some hope for the future.

The medical therapy of primary open-angle glaucoma, like many disorders elsewhere in the body, is directed against the manifestations and not the cause of the disease. While adequate reduction of intraocular pressure appears to retard further visual damage in most individuals, there are a number of perplexing patients in whom progressive damage occurs despite low intraocular pressures. Progress is being made, however, with respect to drug therapy. Of note, re-evaluation of carbonic anhydrase inhibitors suggests the efficacy of lower doses (8). On a more basic level, experiments show that pilocarpine has little effect on monkey eyes with disinserted ciliary muscles (16), a reaffirmation of its mode of action, and more importantly, certain agents such as cytochalasin B may act directly on the trabecular meshwork to reduce outflow resistance (17), possibly by altering microfilaments. What a superb model in which to look for new antiglaucoma agents!

New agents are on the horizon. The β-adrenergic blocking agents seem very promising. Timolol is a β-blocker that appears to reduce intraocular pressure after single and multiple dosing with little or no toxicity (23). Many investigators are evaluating this compound at the present time. The action of timolol appears to be greater than pilocarpine or epinephrine and additive to these drugs. The adrenergic agonists also reduce intraocular pressure, an apparent paradox. These may act via the secondary messenger system of cyclic nucleotides (21). Because epinephrine penetrates the eye so poorly and because many well-controlled glaucoma patients must discontinue this medication due to development of intolerable local and systemic side-effects, congeners of epinephrine with more favorable characteristics are being sought. Dipivalyl epinephrine (DPE) is such an agent that was developed as a lipophilic prodrug of epinephrine, one that would penetrate the cornea easily and be converted to the parent compound once inside the eye. By employing this epinephrine compound in low, effective doses, one would anticipate that extraocular side-effects would be minimized. DPE in very low concentrations, 0.025% - 0.25%, apparently reduces intraocular pressure in short-term and long-term clinical trials (15) with few toxic side-effects. DPE enters the human eye 10 - 20 times more readily than epinephrine and is almost completely converted into the parent compound (13). DPE also stimulates the production of AMP in aqueous humor. Thus, here is an example of a drug developed on the basis of theory to produce certain effects by a predictable mode of action that subsequently was proven, a marvelous example to follow.

Glaucoma investigators are hampered by the lack of an appropriate animal model. Efforts must be channeled in this direction. The recent description of a beagle glaucoma model (9) offers hope for better drug testing. However, with respect to studies of etiology, no animal model of primary open-angle glaucoma is presently known.

Finally, one would be remiss not to mention a major therapeutic problem, compliance. Primary open-angle glaucoma produces little ocular discomfort or immediate disability, while its treatment often does. It is therefore not surprising that there is little reinforcement to induce the patient to continue treatment. Poor compliance to glaucoma therapy, assessed by an interview technique, occurs in about one-third of patients (22). Poor compliance correlates with poor office attendance and normal vision. Physicians routinely underestimate the rate of poor compliance in their own patients. The extensive literature on the management of glaucoma pales in significance when viewed in this perspective. One method to improve compliance in glaucoma therapy would be a device that slowly releases the medication during 4 - 6 months and is inserted by the ophthalmologist at the time of follow-up visits.

Many problems and questions for future research relate to surgical manipulations. Many of the reasons for success or failure of a filtering procedure are unknown. How large should a sclerostomy be? When it fails, what is the nature of the occlusion? Scarring down of episcleral tissue and conjuctiva to the sclerostomy site certainly plays a role. How can scarring and failure be prevented? How important is the composition of the aqueous humor or episcleral tissue in the functioning of the bleb? Does previous medical therapy influence the success of the filtering procedure? Do filtering operations work less frequently in one race versus another? Are experimental valve setons or laser techniques useful? Does surgery prevent progression of field loss? Investigation into these and other questions will improve our results of surgical control of primary open-angle glaucoma until we learn enough to attack the cause of the disease directly.

In conclusion, progress has been made in certain facets of the primary open-angle glaucoma problem. Further advances depend upon new information derived from basic scientific endeavors.

Acknowledgement

Some of the thoughts herein are derived from the chapter "Primary glaucomas" by KRUPIN and PODOS (18).

References

(1) Anderson, D.R.; Hendrickson, A.: Effect of intraocular pressure on rapid axoplasmic transport in monkey optic nerve. Invest. Ophthalmol. 13, 771 (1974)

(2) Becker, B.; Hahn, K.A.: Topical corticosteroids and heredity in primary open-angle glaucoma. Am. J. Ophthalmol. 57, 543 (1964)

(3) Becker, B.; Shin, D.H.: Response to topical epinephrine, a practical prognostic test in patients with ocular hypertension. Arch. Ophthalmol. 94, 2057 (1976)

(4) Bigger, J.F.; Palmberg, P.F.; Zink, H.A.: In vitro corticosteroid: Correlation response with primary open-angle glaucoma and ocular corticosteroid sensitivity. Am. J. Ophthalmol. 79 92 (1975)

(5) Comroe, J.H. jr.; Dripps, R.D.: Scientific basis for the support of biomedical science. Science 192, 105 (1976)

(6) Fankhauser, F.; Spahr, J.; Bebie, H.: Some aspects of the automation of perimetry. Surv. Ophthalmol. 22, 131 (1977)

(7) Francois, J.: Corticosteroid glaucoma. Ann. Ophthalmol. 9 1075 (1977)

(8) Friedland, B.R.; Mallonee, J.; Anderson, D.R.: Short-term dose response characteristics of acetazolamide in man. Arch. Ophthalmol. 95, 1809 (1977)

(9) Gelatt, K.N.; Peiffer, R.L.; Gwin, R.M.; Sauk, J.J. jr.: Glaucomas in the beagle. Trans. Am. Acad. Ophthalmol. Otolaryngol 81, 636 (1976)

(10) Goldmann, H.: Transfer of fluorescein from blood vessels to disc tissue: the theory. Invest. Ophthalmol. 12, 475 (1973)

(11) Graham, P.A.: Epidemiology of simple glaucoma and ocular hypertension. Br. J. Ophthalmol. 56 223 (1972)

(12) Harbin, T.S. jr.; Podos, S.M.; Kolker, A.E.; Becker, B.: Visual field progression in open-angle glaucoma patients presenting with monocular field loss. Trans. Am. Acad. Ophthalmol. Otolaryngol 81, 253 (1976)

(13) Hayreh, S.S.; Revie, I.H.S.; Edwards, J.: Vasogenic origin of visual field defects and optic nerve changes in glaucoma. Br. J. Ophthalmol. 54, 461 (1970)

(14) Johnstone, M.A.; Grant, W.M.: Pressure-dependent changes in structures of the aqueous outflow system of human and monkey eyes. Am. J. Ophthalmol. 75, 365 (1973)

(15) Kaback, M.D.; Podos, S.M.; Harbin, T.S. jr.; Mandell, A.; Becker, B.: The effects of dipivalyl epinephrine on the eye. Am. J. Ophthalmol. 81, 768 (1976)

(16) Kaufman, P.L.; Bárány, E.H.: Loss of acute pilocarpine effect on outflow facility following surgical disinsertion and retrodisplacement of the ciliary muscle from the scleral spur in the cynomolgus monkey. Invest. Ophthalmol. 15 793 (1976)

(17) Kaufman, P.L.: Drugs and the trabecular meshwork. Invest. Ophthalmol. 16, 475 (1977)

(18) Krupin, T.; Podos, S.M.: Primary glaucomas. In: Glaucoma, conceptions of a disease. Heilmann, K., Richardson, K.T. (eds.). Stuttgart: Thieme 1978

(19) Mandell, A.I.; Stentz, F.; Kitabchi, A.E.: A new therapeutic prodrug for the treatment of glaucoma, dipivalyl epinephrine (DPE). Meeting of the American Academy of Ophthalmology and Otolaryngology. Dallas 1977

(20) Nesterov, A.P.: Role of the blockade of Schlemm's canal in pathogenesis of primary open-angle glaucoma. Am. J. Ophthalmol. 70, 691 (1970)

(21) Neufeld, A.H.; Jampol, L.M.; Sears, M.L.: Cyclic AMP in the aqueous humor: the effects of adrenergic agents. Exp. Eye Res. 14, 242 (1972)

(22) Spaeth, G.L.: Visual loss in a glaucoma clinic, I. Sociological considerations. Invest. Ophthalmol. 9, 73 (1970)

(23) Zimmerman, T.J.; Kaufman, H.E.: Timolol: dose-response and duration of action. Arch. Ophthalmol. 95, 605 (1977)

Discussion

LEYDHECKER: I wish to congratulate Dr. PODOS on his excellent survey. In my opinion, the most important objects for clinical research in the near future are the further development of a computer-assisted perimetric quick test, with an instrument that is not too expensive. A fundus camera for the documentation of the optic disk without dilating the pupil is evidently on its way. We urgently need means to predict the tension tolerance, which seems to be impossible at present. We very much wish to understand the drug adaptation mechanism, which is one of the main problems in medical management of glaucomas, especially in β-blocker therapy. It would be most valuable to know the cause and prevention of Tenon's cicatrization after filtering surgery. It would also be fine if we had a means of recording the intraocular pressure continously over the 24 h without disturbing the patient. It would also be good to have means of making the compliance of the patient better.

SAMPAOLESI: In relation to the indication of therapeutics, we do not give more miotics in pigmentary glaucoma because we produced two retinal detachments. We observed in 80% of the cases of pigmentary glaucoma two things: 1) There is a detachment of the anterior hyaloid membrane. The detachment of the hyaloid is responsible for the iridodonesis that we see in these cases. 2) Degeneration in the peripheral retina. These two characteristics give rise to a high frequency of retinal detachments in these patients.

MISHIMA: The point brought up by Dr. SAMPAOLESI (pilocarpine side-effects) indicates the importance of proper dosing. Consideration on the drug delivery is along this line. For this purpose, basic studies on the drug behavior in the eye are needed to give a logical basis to the drug therapy.

HERSCHLER: I would like to suggest that we may be overlooking a very important area of research if we do not explore the biologic and biochemical make-up of the aqueous humor. Some preliminary work I have done using an in vitro model of inhibitory effect on conjunctival fibroblasts in tissue culture would seem to suggest that there is a difference between glaucoma patients and normals in regard to this variable.

LEE: I fully agree with Dr. HERSCHLER's statement about the importance of aqueous humor studies. I believe re-evaluation on aqueous humor concentration utilizing newer microanalysis procedures is essential and a very important parameter in future glaucoma research. For example, utilizing Dr. LAM's microanalysis technique, we have observed that aqueous ascorbate concentration is higher in the eyes with primary open-angle glaucoma than in the eyes with senile cataract or in the eyes with early stage of primary angle-closure glaucoma.

FRANÇOIS: I think that in the future research in the glaucoma field should especially involve the study of the metabolism and of the enzymes in the trabecular meshwork and in the aqueous humor. This is what we are now trying to do.

DRANCE: Dr. PODOS very kindly mentioned that we showed that glaucoma surgery does not influence the progression. However, our studies have shown that not all patients whose pressures are operatively controlled do not progress.

LAMGHAM: The site of increased resistance in the glaucomatous eye is basic to programs of glaucoma research. Until this problem is resolved, there is the danger that biochemical, enzymatic, and morphologic studies on the trabecular meshwork may have little, if any, relevance to prevention of glaucoma. In this respect, there is significant evidence that the intrascleral channels where blood and aqueous humor meet is the site of maximal outflow resistance in both normal and glaucomatous eyes. The adrenergic agonists and modulators acting on blood flow to the ciliary processes and to the intra- and episcleral system provide a means of bringing the pressure of glaucomatous eyes to normal. Unfortunately, with continued treatment, the intraocular pressure response decreases. In my view, it is of major importance to clarify the adrenoceptor mechanisms causing this tachyphylaxis.

Advances in Ocular Pharmacology

Irving H. Leopold

University of California, California College of Medicine, Department of Ophthalmology, Irvine, Cal. 92717, USA

Within the past decade, considerable pharmacologic advances have occurred that potentially influence ophthalmologic functions, disease, and practice.

Adrenergic Agents

A variety of agents acting through the adrenergic system have been found to favorably influence the intraocular pressure. The β-blocking agents are currently in vogue. Most of these β-blockers have a significant effect on systemic blood pressure. When administered orally, agents such as propranolol, practolol, atenolol, pindolol, timolol, nadalol, bupranolol, metoprolol, and oxyprenolol will not only lower systemic blood pressure but will also lower intraocular pressure. Most of these have been demonstrated to lower intraocular pressure when topically applied to the eye. In the ensuing years much will be written and presented concerning these agents, for they all appear to be helpful in inducing hypotension in eyes with glaucoma and ocular hypertension.

The side-effects of these agents are varied. Not all produce local anesthesia in the cornea as seen with propranolol. Not all produce a dry eye syndrome as seen with practolol and possibly metoprolol. Some produce bradycardia and systemic hypotension when topically applied as well as bronchospasm, noticeably in asthmatics. A forerunner of these agents, pronethalol induced tumor growth in experimental animals. Some of the more recent agents appear to also have this action. The mechanism for the fall of intraocular pressure after topical administration has not been clarified. It appears that receptor blockage of both β_1 and β_2 is not essential for the ocular hypotensive effect, as atenolol, a β_1-blocker, essentially also lowers intraocular pressure in effective fashion.

These agents have the advantage of not inducing ciliary spasm, pupillary constriction, and usually require only twice daily application to control the diurnal fluctuations. They also appear to work in co-operation with other hypotensive agents such as pilocarpine, epinephrine, and acetazolamide. The actions of each of the β-blockers may differ in several ways. Human trials and experience over time may permit proper selection of the most effective and least hazardous of the numerous β-blocking agents.

Labetalol is a β-blocking agent that also possesses α-adrenergic blocking ability. This property distinguishes it from all other β-blocking agents currently under investigation. It lowers pressure when topically applied in narrow-angle as well as open-angle glaucoma.

There is clinical evidence that labetalol may be safer than β-blocking agents for asthmatic patients. It seems less likely to cause bronchoconstriction than available β-blockers. It does not affect heart rate.

Some of the data accumulated by PODOS, LEOPOLD, MURRAY, and WEI shows the marked hypotensive effect of this agent on intraocular pressure in experimental studies. The dose-response curves are impressive. The peak effect occurred approximately 30 - 60 min after a dose of 1% and persisted for 6 h.

There is some evidence that this drug binds to melanin and particularly in the pigmentary epithelium of the eye. The animal data to date suggests reversibility of this finding. There are no comparable studies of melanin binding of the other β-blockers, atenolol or timolol, as yet. It will be important to monitor retinal and particularly macular function in all of the patients exposed to these drugs. However, studies by POYNTER, MARTIN, HARRISON, and COOK failed to reveal any evidence of ocular toxicity by detailed ophthalmologic and histologic examination carried out on rats, rabbits, cats, and dogs, even after 7 months of continuous systemic therapy with labetalol. This is certainly a provocative agent for potential use in ophthalmology. The systemic use of β-blocking agents for control of glaucoma seems to be gaining support.

β-Agonists have been known to lower intraocular pressure by reduction of aqueous formation. In recent years new agonists have been evaluated. These include salbutamol, a new catecholamine with selective β_2-agonist properties.

Isoproterenol never achieved wide-scale use because of local hyperemia and cardiovascular side-effects. Salbutamol in 4% concentration produces a marked hyperemia and irritation. It is quite possible that a prodrug derivative of isoproterenol might avoid some of these side-effects and make this a useful agent, particularly if the prodrug could avoid the local irritation as well as the cardiac stimulation. Experimental studies by KASS and co-workers and MURRAY and co-workers have shown a significant drop in pressure with dipivalyl isoproterenol without the cardiovascular effect. This requires confirmation through human experience.

The racemic form of isoproterenol has been studied. It is possible that, by using the dextroisomer only, one could produce a greater reduction in intraocular pressure than with the racemic mixture of the dextro- and levoisomers. This dextroisomer appears to be free of the cardiac effect in experimental animals. Isoxuprine and nylidrine are also β-agonists and lower intraocular pressure in 1% solution. Pargyline, an inhibitor of monamine oxidase in 0.5% concentration, has been shown to lower intraocular pressure.

For years epinephrine has been the mainstay of the adrenergic agents in the therapy of open-angle glaucoma. With the use of gonioscopy, it was possible to separate patients into open- and narrow-angle glaucoma and avoid the unfortunate rises in intraocular pressure formerly seen in eyes with occludable angles following epinephrine. Studies in recent years have shown that doses as low as 0.6% produced statistically significant changes in intraocular pressure. No change in the outflow facility was noted until the drug concentration of 1% epinephrine was reached. Further increases to 2% failed to produce any additional improvement. The data suggest that two different populations of receptors may be involved in the epinephrine-induced type of effect. One set of receptors activated at low doses may affect the aqueous production. A second set of receptors activated by concentrations of 1% epinephrine resulted in increased outflow.

Years of experience have shown that the side-effects of the use of topical epinephrine are numerous. Most annoying is the high incidence of conjuctival reactions ranging from hyperemia to severe allergic conjunctivitis. Sears' data show that the incidence of side-effects of this type ranges from 10% - 50% and appear to increase with prolonged use.

Recently, a new drug, dipivalyl epinephrine, has become available. This dipivalyl attachment to the epinephrine molecule makes it a prodrug. It has to be broken down by the ocular tissues and fluids before it can act as free epinephrine. The application of the prodrug to the surface of the eyes may have the advantages of reducing considerably the amount of free epinephrine available to produce the red-eye syndrome. Data presented by MANDEL in 1976 and recently by YABLONSKI, SHIN, KOLKER, KASS, and BECKER make this seem an exciting possibility for this agent in that there is marked reduction in the red-eye syndrome upon the use of this effective hypotensive agent. It appears to give all the benefits of epinephrine but at lower concentrations and with some markedly reduced side-effects. Animal experimentation showed that it has a less likelihood of producing cardiovascular symptoms. This also appears to be substantiated in humans.

The irritation produced in patients by epinephrine and the intolerance of patients for its continued use has stimulated a re-evaluation for other known adrenergic compounds. Norepinephrine has been shown by POLLACK to be effective in lowering intra ocular pressure. POLLACK and ROSSI found that norepinephrine produced conjunctival hyperemia in many patients; however, there was an absence of cardiac stimulation with norepinephrine as compared to epinephrine. One patient in POLLACK's studies showed an allergic reaction to epinephrine that cleared promptly when norepinephrine was substituted.

Norepinephrine, the adrenergic neurotransmitter, decreases the resistance to aqueous outflow and thereby reduced intraocular pressure.

Agents that deplete the catecholamines from the endings of the sympathetic nerve fibers such as guanethidine and 6-hydroxydopanine allow the end organ receptors to be sensitized to epinephrine. Guanethidine alone topically and systemically administered can lower intraocular pressure on glaucomatous, hypertensive, and normotensive eyes. Long-term clinical trials with guanethidine and epinephrine have substantiated the effectiveness of such combinations in cases of glaucoma not controlled in traditional maximal therapy.

New information is available on the cholenergic agents such as new forms of pilocarpine, aceclydine compounds such as oxytremorine, and new delivery systems. Carbonic anhydrase inhibitors are under study for improvement in dosage and schedules. Variations of hydrocannabinols for topical and systemic use offer promise.

Mechanism of Adrenergic Treatment of Glaucoma

Marvin L. Sears

Yale University, School of Medicine, 333 Cedar Street, New Haven, Conn. 06510, USA

Effects of Topical Epinephrine

The pressure-lowering effects of adrenergic drugs applied topically to the human eye are complex and varied, but at least three phases have been described: 1) an early decrease in pressure that appears to be related both to a decrease in aqueous inflow and an increased outflow; 2) a second phase of increased outflow lasting several hours; 3) a late, progressive increase in outflow even days, weeks, and months after therapy.

Early Effects

Minutes after administration of topical epinephrine, the eye first becomes white, α-adrenergic effects (vasoconstriction and mydriasis) predominate, and possibly a fall in ciliary blood flow occurs. Studies of fluorescein turnover in the human eye, after topical epinephrine indicated that the initial reduction in intraocular pressure was a consequence of decreased inflow of aqueous. Tonographic studies done in the 1950s suggested that not all the reduction in intraocular pressure could be explained in this manner. More recent tonographic studies of this early effect showed an increased outflow shortly after a single topical dose of epinephrine that could last hours longer. The early decrease is, in part, actually a pseudofacility, i.e., a decrease in the pressure-dependent part of aqueous inflow. (Tonography measures gross facility only). The remainder of the increase in gross facility is probably an increase in true facility of outflow, similar to the effect after degeneration release of norepinephrine.

If part of the increase in outflow is in reality a decrease in (the pressure-sensitive part of) aqueous humor formation, how might this effect occur? The aqueous humor is formed by a process of ultrafiltration and secretion across the blood-aqueous barrier. In all likelihood these two processes are at least linked in series. The first step in the formation of aqueous humor is the development of a plasma filtrate in the stroma of the ciliary processes by "ultrafiltration" across the fenestrated capillary wall. The ciliary epithelia act upon this stromal pool. Although there are no nerves within the epithelial layers of the ciliary processes, α-adrenergic receptors are probably present in the vessels of the stroma to mediate vasoconstriction. Limiting the plasma filtrate entering the ciliary stroma by vasoconstriction, before it is acted upon by the epithelia, will decrease formation (inflow occurring through ultrafiltration) and appear as an increase in total facility with manometric or tonographic techniques. A direct effect on true facility of outflow at this stage would also be α-mediated because the eye still manifests other α-adrenergic effects: mydriasis and vasoconstriction. There is considerable pharmacologic data to support α influences upon outflow (5).

Intermediate Effects

After topical epinephrine, an increase in outflow, intermediate in onset, almost certainly represents an increase in true facility. This second phase of increased outflow lasts many hours after topical epinephrine. Although an early α-mediated increase in true outflow facility may occur, but hours after topical epinephrine, an increased outflow persists at a time when the eye is no longer white (from vasoconstriction) and the pupil no longer dilated. These intermediate effects, at least in part, probably involve the production of c-AMP. In the rabbit, changes in c-AMP in the aqueous humor, possibly a reflection of intracellular events, have been used to correlate the effect of adrenergic agents with changes of intraocular pressure. Topically administered epinephrine increases c-AMP in the aqueous humor, the increase persists more than 5 h, and it can be prevented by appropriate antagonists. Further, smaller decrements in intraocular pressure after epinephrine from extended daily treatment are accompanied by smaller increases in c-AMP in the aqueous humor. On the other hand, under conditions of sympathetic denervation, an exaggerated decrease in intraocular pressure and increase in outflow after epinephrine is accompanied by an increase in the c-AMP content of the aqueous humor. The increase in outflow facility and c-AMP production are both two to three times normal in the supersensitive eye. Finally, a two- to threefold increase in outflow is seen after direct intracameral injection of c-AMP in a final molar concentration (anterior chamber) of 2×10^{-4}M. Some analogues are even more potent. The progressive late increase in outflow, after topical epinephrine, originally described by BALLINTINE (1), was confirmed in other clinics. The mechanism has been discussed previously. Recently in our laboratory, Dr. HAYASAKA has shown that epinephrine can activate lysosomal hyaluronidase derived from iris tissue (3). The activation is independent of AMP production and is not produced by precursors or metabolites of the hormone. Of course, our thinking has been that the late increase in outflow facility seen after topical epinephrine may be mediated via a reduction in that part of the resistance provided by hyaluronidase-sensitive mucopolysaccharide. Whether this explanation is valid for the human eye is not yet known.

Adrenergic Effects on Inflow

Dr. GREGORY and Dr. BAUSHER of our laboratory have done a careful kinetic study of adenyl cyclase activity using a washed particulate fraction of homogenates of rabbit ciliary processes. The particulate fraction is maximally stimulated by β-active catecholamines. Guanyl cyclase activity has been found at about one-half that of adenylate cyclase. Its role has not been completely worked out. These investigators also found AMP phosphodiesterase, with about two times as much activity as adenyl cyclase in the particulate fraction and about 20 times as much in the (3000 × g centrifugation) supernatant. Two kinetically distinct c-AMP phosphodisterases have been found.

In vivo pressure studies conducted in 1974 in our laboratory have shown that timolol (6), a potent β-antagonist, reduces intraocular pressure in rabbits whose outflow facility is compromised. Recently, photofluorimetric studies have indicated that timolol reduces intraocular pressure by decreasing aqueous inflow. Thus, it seems that β-stimulation (2, 4) and blockade (7) both cause significant reductions in intraocular pressure, and, in all likelihood, working on aqueous inflow.

Timolol

The pharmacologic profile of timolol resembles that described for other β-adrenergic blocking agents, such as propranolol and sotalol. Timolol was studied as the l-isomer, as the hydrogen maleate salt. It has no apparent effect on pupillary diameter and does not influence ciliary body tone sufficiently to cause refractive change. Consequently, it may have a special place in the treatment of young glaucoma patients or in those with cataractous changes in whom acuity is adversely affected by miosis. The effects of 0.1% - 0.5% timolol given twice a day for up to more than 2 years to patients with ocular hypertension or open-angle glaucoma has been studied. The drug has been generally well-tolerated, with a minimum of side-effects. Details have been given by others at this seminar.

At the moment we believe that timolol may reduce inflow but not by its potent β-adrenergic blocking mechanism. Our reasoning is as follows. Determining K_Is for certain adrenergic blocking agents as propranolol, pindolol, timolol, Dr. GREGORY indicates that while the binding and blocking potencies parallel each other, the pressure-lowering effect of timolol appears to be more marked than pindolol, for example, although inhibition of epinephrine-stimulated adenyl cyclase activity for these two compounds is quite similar. Further studies will be required to solve the puzzling problems raised by the apparently similar effect of both β-agonists and antagonists on aqueous inflow.

References

(1) Ballintine, E.J.: In: Glaucoma. Transactions of the 5 Conference. Newell, F.W. (ed.). New York: Josiah Macy 1960

(2) Eakins, K.E.: Effect of intravitreous injections of norepinephrine epinephrine, and isoproterenol on the intraocular pressure and aqueous humor dynamics of rabbit eyes. J. Pharmacol. Exp. Ther. 140, 79 (1963)

(3) Hayasaka, S.; Sears, M.L.: Effects of epinephrine, indomethacin, acetylsalicylic acid, dexamethasone, and cyclic AMP on the in vitro activity of lysosomal hyaluronidase from the rabbit iris. Invest. Ophthalmol. Vis. Sci. (in press) (1978)

(4) Sears, M.L.: Catecholamines in relation to the eye. In: Handbook of physiology: Endocrinology VI. Astwood, E., Creep, R. (eds.), Chapter 35. pp. 553-590. American Physiological Society.

(5) Sears, M.L.: Perspectives in glaucoma research. Invest. Ophthalmol. Vis. Sci. 17, 6 (1978) (Friedenwald lecture)

(6) Vareilles, P.; Silverstone, D.; Plazonnet, B.; LeDouarec, J.-C.; Sears, M.L.; Stone, C.A.: Comparison of the effects of Timolol and other adrenergic agents on intraocular pressure in the rabbit. Invest. Ophthalmol. Vis. Csi. 16, 987 (1977)

(7) Yablonski, M.E.; Zimmerman, T.J.; Waltman, S.R.; Becker, B.: A fluorophotometric study of the effect of topical Timolol on aqueous humor dynamics. Exp. Eye Res. (in press) (1978)

Discussion

ZIMMERMAN: First, I would like to thank Dr. LEOPOLD for his excellent summary of some of the new ocular hypotensive drugs that are being tested. I would also like to echo Dr. LEOPOLD's feeling that we should continue to look for other β-blockers in the hope of finding one that might be superior in some way to timolol. Finally, I would like to thank Dr. LEOPOLD for pointing out that all new drugs should be thoroughly tested for side-effects in controlled studies before they are released to the public.

ZIMMERMAN: As Dr. LEOPOLD pointed out in his paper, the β-blockers are not only exciting clinically but also for their basic research potential. As for the mechanism of action of the β-blockers, it has recently been shown in two separate independent studies that timolol decreases the rate of aqueous secretion in men. These were single drop studies and showed that the decrease in the rate of aqueous secretion totally accounted for the accompanying decrease in intraocular pressure. I was pleased to see that you found similar results in the rabbit. I agree that the ciliary epithelium is the most likely place to begin the search.

LEYDHECKER: In my patients I could not see an increased effect of epinephrine in long-term use.

Effects of Adrenergic Drugs on the Eye: Some Experimental Studies

Saiichi Mishima, Tadashi Tamura, Masahiro Takase, Shigetoshi Nagataki

University of Tokyo, School of Medicine, Department of Ophthalmology, 7-3-1 Hongo, Bunkyo-Ku, Tokyo-113 Japan

This paper summarizes some of the experimental results obtained at our department concerning the effects of adrenergic drugs on the eye.

Effects of Bupranolol Hydrochloride on the Intraocular Pressure (IOP) in Human Eyes

Bupranolol hydrochloride, a β-adrenergic blocker, lowered the IOP in normal volunteers and glaucoma patients without significant changes in the pupil diameter and refraction (7). A dose-response study was carried out in a total of 30 patients, 12 with ocular hypertension and 18 with primary open-angle glaucoma, comprising 14 males and 16 females aged 21 - 65 years. In each individual, 35 μl of bupranolol solution was instilled in one eye and the fellow eye served as the control; 0.2%, 0.5%, and 1.0% solutions were tested at appropriate intervals. Applanation tonometry was carried out every hour after instillation in both eyes. The IOP before instillation was similar in both eyes, being within the range of 20 - 30 mm Hg. The peak hypotensive effects were obtained about 2 h after instillation, and the IOP difference between both eyes was plotted against the logarithm of concentrations (Fig. 1). An extrapolation of the dose-response relationship yielded a least effective concentration of 0.13 ± 0.049% (SD).

The effect duration was defined as the time between the peak effect and the termination of the hypotensive effect. The effect durations were plotted against the logarithm of concentrations (Fig. 2). The relationship was linear and an extrapolation of the regression line intersected with the concentration axis at 0.16 ± 0.049%. This agrees well with the least effective concentration obtained above. The slope of the regression line was $0.2 \pm 0.044\ h^{-1}$: this was termed as "the rate of effect disappearance."

After instillation, drugs are rapidly taken up by the cornea and then released slowly into the anterior chamber, whereupon quick distribution to the iris and ciliary body occurs (6). Since the drug concentration in the tears is reduced to a negligible level in 10 min, subsequent intraocular drug kinetics can be simulated by a two-compartment open model. The anterior chamber concentration changes are approximated by a biexponential equation, and after the peak time the concentration decreases in an exponential manner. An analysis (10) of the pupil responses to

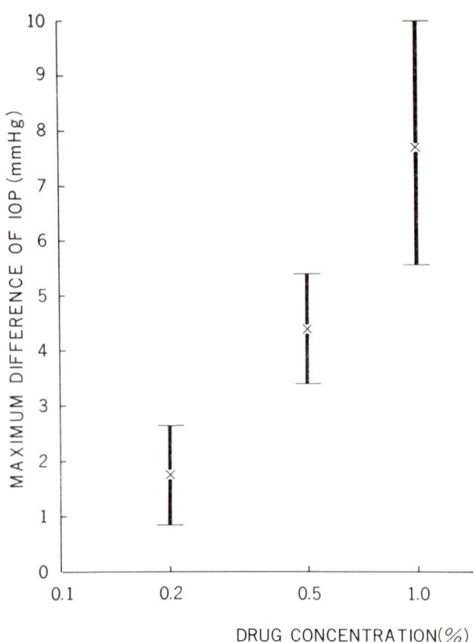

Fig. 1. The maximum IOP effects and the logarithm of bupranolol concentrations. Mean ± SD of 30 cases are shown.

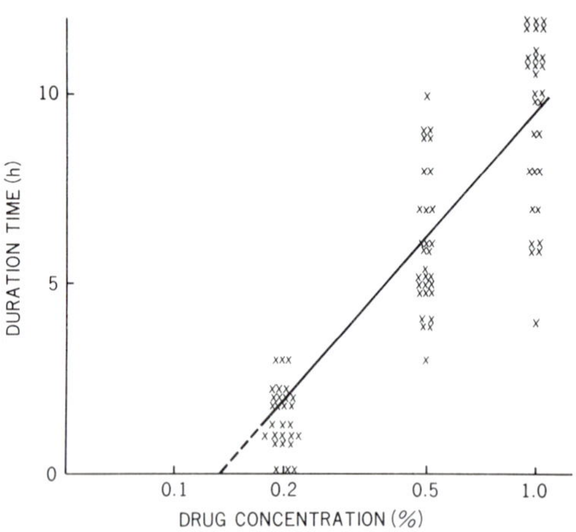

Fig. 2. The relation between the logarithm of bupranolol concentration and the duration of the hypotensive effects.

miotic and mydriatic drugs showed that the above kinetics hold true for the human eye, and the rate constant of drug elimination was calculated for various drugs.

The durations of miotic and mydriatic effects, defined in a similar way as above, were shown to be related linearly with the logarithm of drug concentrations, the slope of the regression line agreed with the rate constant of drug elimination, and the extrapolation of the line gave the least effective concentration (10). This procedure was supported by the theory of LEVY (4) concerning the pharmacokinetics of drug responses.

The present analysis of the hypotensive responses was carried out in analogy to the above. However, since the mechanism and time relationship between the intraocular drug concentration and the hypotensive effects are not known, we adopted the term "the rate of effect disappearance." The pharmacologic basis of this concept is still obscure, but it is hoped that this parameter will aid us in the study of pharmacokinetics of antiglaucomatous drug.

Aqueous Humor Dynamics in Man

The conventional tonography was performed on both eyes of 23 patients selected from the patients described above, in a random order of laterality 2 h after instillation of 1% bupranolol solution in one eye (7). The aqueous flow rate was calculated assuming the episcleral venous pressure to be 10 mm Hg. The results are shown in Table 1; a significant decrease in the flow rate was obtained after instillations.

Table 1. Tonography 1 h before and 2 h after bupranolol instillation

	Before		After	
	Treated	Control	Treated	Control
Outflow facility $\mu l\ min^{-1}\ mm\ Hg^{-1}$	0.12±0.038[a]	0.14±0.028	0.14±0.028	0.15±0.047
Aqueous flow rate $\mu l\ min^{-1}$	1.70±0.39	1.78±0.38	1.09±0.30	1.80±0.33

[a] Mean ± SD of 23 cases

Use of fluorescein permits investigation into aqueous humor dynamics in man. Among various methods (1, 3, 5), Jones and MAURICES' method (3) was used to calculate k_0 because of its simplicity and safety in fluorescein application. Twenty microliters of 2% l-epinephrine bitartarate or 1% bupranolol was instilled in one eye of 11 normal male volunteers, between 21 and 33 years of age. One hour later, 20 μl of 10% fluorescein was instilled in both eyes, the concentration changes of fluorescein in the cornea and anterior chamber were measured with an objective fluorophotometer, and k_0 was calculated. At the end of the experiment, the IOP and the anterior chamber depth were measured. The results are given in Table 2; a significant reduction in k_0 was found after instillation without change in the anterior chamber depth. The value of k_0 is the sum of k_{dpa} and k_{fa}. Since our previous study (5) showed that the ratio k_{dpa}/k_{fa} was 0.095, the reduction in k_0 exceeding 10% after epinephrine and bupranolol could not be attributed to decrease of k_{dpa} alone and was considered to be due to reduction in the aqueous flow rate. As for the epinephrine effect, this agrees with the statement of GOLDMANN (2). The amount of reduction in k_0 after bupranolol was, however, less than that obtained by tonography. This method averaged the drug effects over several hours, whereas the tonography was performed at the peak of the drug effects.

Table 2. Effects of epinephrine and bupranolol on aqueous humor dynamics and the anterior chamber depth of 11 normal volunteers

	k_0 ($x\ 10^2\ min^{-1}$)	IOP (mm Hg)	Anterior chamber depth (mm)
2% epinephrine	1.1 ± 0.15[a]	12 ± 1.9	3.65 ± 0.32
1% bupranolol	1.2 ± 0.13	13 ± 1.8	3.9 ± 0.17
Control	1.35 ± 0.14	13 ± 1.7	3.8 ± 0.28

[a] Mean ± SD

Effects on the Ultrastructure of the Ciliary Epithelium of the Rabbit

Two percent dl-isoproterenol, 5% salbutamol, or 2% l-norepinephrine were instilled in one eye of rabbits, and the non pigmented epithelium of the iridial and ciliary processes was examined with an electron microscope (8). Most significant changes were found in the non pigmented epithelia 20 min after instillation of isoproterenol or salbutamol. The changes embraced a marked increase in smooth endoplasmic reticulum (SER), free ribosomes, diffuse particles of the nucleus, and enlargement of the ciliary channels (Fig.3).

The ciliary epithelial cells were classified into SER-poor and SER-rich cells (Fig. 4). Through survey of 40 - 100 non pigmented epithelial cells, the incidence of SER-rich cells was calculated. Twenty minutes after isoproterenol instillation, the incidence significantly increased and was more pronounced in the iridial than in the ciliary process (Fig.5). Similary, salbutamol caused a marked increase in the incidence 20 min after instillation. With both drugs the cells with highly developed SER (Fig.4), which were never encountered in the normal ciliary epithelia, were found abundantly. After instillation of norepinephrine, no change occurred in the cytoplasmic organelles of the ciliary epithelia. Pretreatment of the animal with intravenous bupranolol (5 mg/kg body weight) 10 min before isoproterenol completely supressed the effects in increasing the SER.

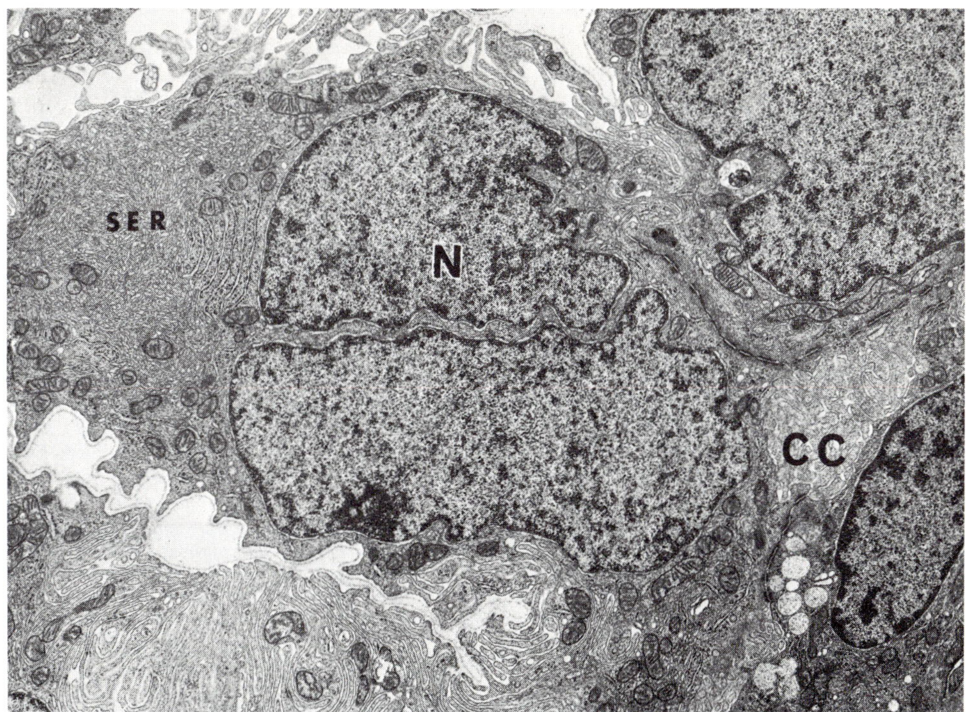

Fig.3. The non pigmented epithelial cell of the ciliary process 20 min after instillation of isoproterenol. A major part of the cytoplasm is occupied by SER and RER. Dense particles in the nucleus are increased and the ciliary channel is dilated containing many microvilli. The bar indicates 1 μm. N, nucleus; cc, ciliary channel.

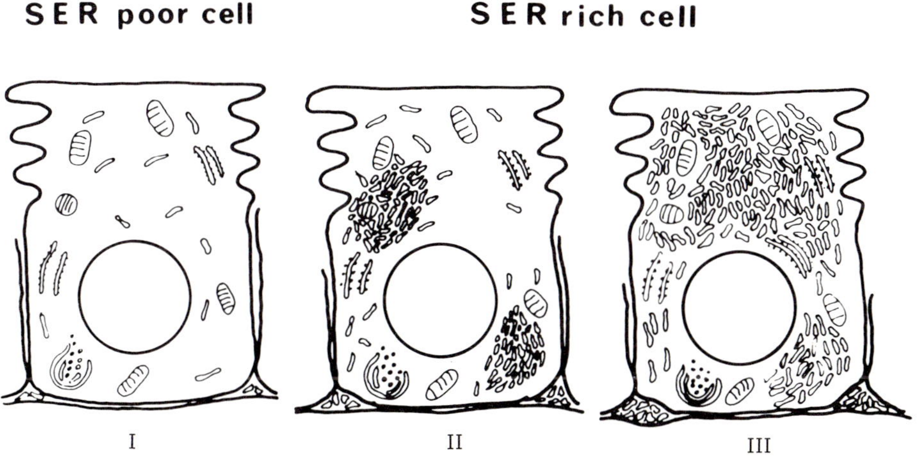

Fig.4. Classification of the non pigmented epithelial cells into three classes. I, SER-poor cell; II, SER-richt cell; III, cells with very highly developed SER, which are found 20 min after isoproterenol or salbutamol instillation.

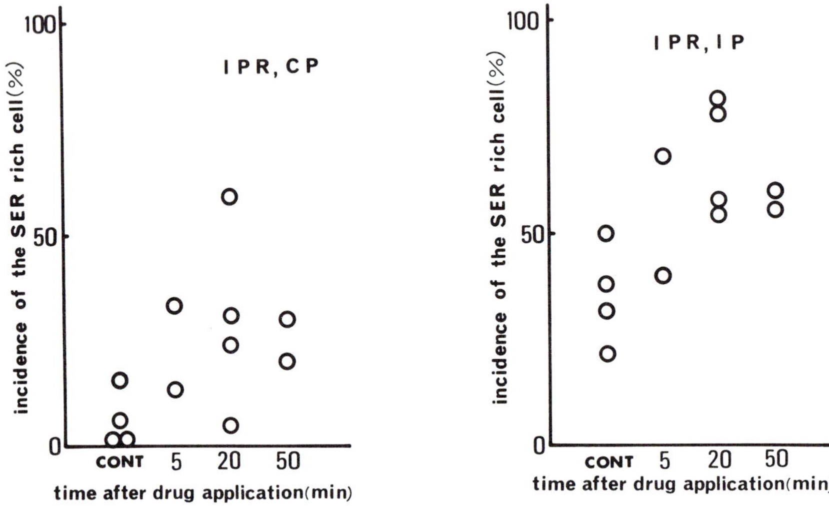

Fig.5. The incidences of the SER-rich cells (a) in the ciliary process after isoproterenol instillation and (b) in the iridial processes after isoproterenol instillation.

These results indicate that β-agonist and blockers have opposite effects on the intracellular organelles, probably on the cellular activity, of the non pigmented epithelia of the ciliary processes. Although dose-response study is required to confirm pharmacoligic effects, the β-adrenergic effects on the ciliary epithelia is interesting in view of the fact that β-blockers reduce aqueous humor formation. In the isolated rabbit ciliary processes, β-adrenergic stimulation increases tissue c-AMP (9). Topical isoproterenol at the dose used in this study also increased c-AMP in the ciliary processes of rabbits (TANURA, unpublished). The relation between these biochemical results and present findings would be an interesting subject of future studies.

References

(1) Goldmann, H.: Abflussdruck, Minutenvolumen und Widerstand der Kammerwasser-Strömung des Menschen. Doc. Ophthalmol. 5, 278-355 (1951)

(2) Goldmann, H.: L'origine de l'hypertension oculaire dans le glaucome primitif. Ann. Oculist. 184, 1086-1105 (1951)

(3) Jones, R.F.; Maurice, D.M.: New methods of measuring the rate of aqueous flow in man with fluorescein. Exp. Eye Res. 5, 208-220 (1966)

(4) Levy, G.; Gibaldi, M.: Pharmacokinetics of drug action. Ann. Rev. Pharmacol. 12, 85-98 (1972)

(5) Nagataki, S.: Aqueous humor dynamics of human eyes as studied using fluorescein. Jpn. J. Ophthalmol. 19, 235-249 (1975)

(6) Sieg, J.W.; Robinson, J.R.: Mechanistic studies on transcorneal permeation of pilocarpine. J. Pharmacol. Sci. 65, 1816-1822 (1976)

(7) Takase, M.; Komuro, S.; Nanba, H.; Araie, M.: Effects of topical bupranolol hydrochrolide on the intraocular pressure. Jpn. J. Ophthalmol. 22, 140-152 (1978)

(8) Ueno, K.; Tamura, T.; Mishima, S.: Effects of adrenergic drugs on the ciliary epithelium of albino rabbits. Metab. Ophthalmol. 1, 199-207 (1977)

(9) Waitzman, M.B.; Woods, W.D.: Some characteristics of an adenyl cyclase preparation from rabbit ciliary process tissue. Exp. Eye Res. 12, 99-111 (1971)

(10) Yoshida, S.; Mishima, S.: A pharmacokinetic analysis of the pupil response to topical pilocarpine and tropicamide. Jpn. J. Ophthalmol. 19, 121-138 (1975).

Discussion

ZIMMERMAN: I simply would like to congratulate you and your group on this excellent contribution. It is work like this that will greatly advance our knowledge concerning the ocular drugs.

ARMALY: Dr. Mishima's comments are equally applicable to both Dr. Drance's data. Did they look at their results for another possible cutoff line, say 6 or 7 or 4 mm Hg. It is important when we attempt to replicate a drug response study that we explore not only the proposed cutoff line or point but look for another possible cutoff line in the data.

LEYDHECKER: Clinically, 4% pilocarpine does not act better than 2%. From one of your Figures, I had the impression that your results showed a longer action of 4% as compared to 2% pilocarpine.

MISHIMA: 1) The pupil response is, we feel, the best index for the study of ocular pharmacokinetics; the changes in the pupil diameter can be converted to a parameter that is proportional to the drug concentration in the iris. In this manner, we demonstrated the time course of pilocarpine concentration in the iris. The method entails calculation of the parameter, $R/(R_{max} - R)$, where R is the response defined as the pupil diameter difference before and after pilocarpine instillations and R_{max} is the maximum response defined as the pupil diameter difference before instillation and the minimum attainable pupil diameter, i.e., 1 mm. It was shown, through in vitro studies on the human sphincter, that this parameter is proportional to pilocarpine concentration in the biophase of the iris sphincter muscles.
Plotting of $\log \frac{R}{R_{max} - R}$ against time gives a biexponentional curve that represents the time course of the pilocarpine concentration changes in the eye. A computer program for the analysis of this curve was developed by NAGATAKI of our department, which enabled us to calculate various parameters of pharmacokinetics. One of these parameters is the rate constant of drug elimination.
The hypotensive effects of pilocarpine are certainly due to the drug in the eye. What is the relation between the pilocarpine concentration changes and the change in the intraocular pressure? I understand that this is what Prof. LEYDHECKER is asking. We do not know the detail of its mechanism or the temporal relationship. For this reason, we called the parameter calculated from the intraocular pressure response the rate of effect disappearance, to distinguish it from the rate constant of drug elimination. We, however, know the concentration changes of pilocarpine in the eye and the effect, i.e., the intraocular pressure changes. We are hoping to construct a computer model to simulate the intraocular pressure response to investigate the relationship you and we are asking for.

The concept of least effective concentration and the rate of effect disappearance is useful clinically, namely, the duration of the effect (T), as defined in the text, is given by the following equation:

$$T = (\ln \frac{C}{Cl})/\alpha$$

where C is the concentration given, Cl is the least effective concentration, and α is the rate of effect disappearance.

2) As regards the effects of 2%, 4%, and 8% pilocarpine, I would like to draw your attention to the basic principle of the dose-response relationship. The relationship between the response and logarithm of concentration has a sigmoid shape and can be regarded to be almost linear between the range of 20% - 80% of the maximum response. Within this range, the response increases as the concentration increases. We may draw a line above this range to show the concentration that can no longer increase the response significantly and call it the maximum effect dose. In the case of pilocarpine, this level is between 2% and 4%, and for this reason concentrations higher than 2% cannot give significantly greater effect. However, the duration of the effect becomes longer for the reasons I described above. The rate constant of pilocarpine elimination is about $0.3\,h^{-1}$ the least effective concentration to the pupil is about 0.15%, and the duration calculated on this basis agrees fairly well with the experience of Dr. DRANCE. With high concentrations, we saturate the effect, and the amount exceeding the maximum effect dose does not contribute to the effect but may be toxic. Pilocarpine is a relatively safe drug, but it has side-effects as pointed out by Prof. SAMPAOLESI. Furthermore, pilocarpine is accumulated in the lens and may be cataractogenic as reported by Levene. We believe that it is important to realize that prolongation of the effect duration by high concentration is at the cost of possible toxicity. We, therefore, prefer to use lower concentration, i.e., 0.5% - 2.0% by repeated applications. A slide is shown to demonstrate the intraocular pilocarpine concentration by a single drop and repeated instillations. In the case of pilocarpine, maintenance of appropriate intraocular concentration is better than the pulse-wise dosing of high concentration. We use 4% pilocarpine occasionally, but never higher than this.

Diurnal Variation of Intraocular Pressure and Its Significance in the Medical Treatment of Primary Open-Angle Glaucoma

Yoshiaki Kitazawa and Takeshi Horie

University of Tokyo, School of Medicine, Department of Ophthalmology
7-3-1 Hongo, Bunkyo-Ku, Tokyo-113, Japan

The knowledge of the diurnal variation of intraocular pressure (IOP) is of importance for the adequate medical therapy of glaucomas and for accurate appraisal of the drug effects on the IOP (1-8). In the previous contributions, we reported on the diurnal fluctuations of IOP measured hourly for 24 h with a Goldmann applanation tonometer in normal subjects, ocular hypertensives, and patients with primary open-angle glaucoma. It was noted that in contrast to most of the previous studies reporting lowest values in the afternoon and highest values in the morning, the IOP was the lowest early in the morning and highest in the daytime in the majority of the subjects studied. In extension of these studies, we attempted to determine the rhythmicity of the diurnal pressure variation by fitting each diurnal curve to a cosine curve by means of the least square method. We found that in the majority of our cases the curves could be represented reasonably well by a cosine curve with a frequency of one cycle in 24 ± 4 h; thus, it was suggested that the diurnal pressure variation is circadian. The above studies indicated two possibilities of clinical importance. One was to predict the peak pressure on the bases of the single measurement of the IOP, which will be of great importance for the installation of the proper medical regimen. The second possibility indicated was to develop a more precise approach to the evaluation of the drug effects on the IOP.

The purpose of the present paper is to report on the results of our study on the diurnal rhythm of the IOP variation and to discuss the above concepts.

Subjects and Methods

Ninety-eight subjects (186 eyes) - 21 normal subjects, 38 ocular hypertensives, and 39 primary open-angle glaucoma patients - were studied. The age of the subjects ranged 12 - 75 years, with a mean age of 41.4 years; 29 were males and 69 were females. All the normal subjects had an IOP of less than 20 mm Hg on repeated measurements with a Goldmann applanation tonometer and no ocular pathology except for minimal refractive errors and/or early senile lenticular change. The diagnosis of the ocular hypertension was made on the basis of applanation tension exceeding 20 mm Hg and the absence of pathologic visual field changes when examined with a Goldmann perimeter. Primary open-angle glaucoma was diagnosed only in the presence of typical glaucomatous visual field changes disclosed by the examination with a Goldmann perimeter and applanation pressure exceeding 20 mm Hg. The IOP was measured every hour for at least 24 h with a Goldmann applanation tonometer. During the daytime, each subject was ambulatory but was asked to be seated quietly for at least 5 prior to each measurement. Subjects stayed in bed during their regular sleeping hours and could sleep between measurements. The first measurement of the day was usually at 11 a.m. Glaucoma patients had their antiglaucoma medications discontinued at least 96 prior to admission. Full 24-h measurements were repeated twice in 12 subjects and three times in four subjects. Altogether, 226 diurnal pressure measurements were performed on 186 eyes. The same examiner made all the tonometric measurements in each subject. The subjects were urged to maintain their regular sleep-wake cycles at least 3 days prior to the study. Although the pattern of sleep-wake cycles varied between individuals, all subjects went to bed around 10 p.m. to midnight and awoke around 6 - 8 a.m.

Results

Prediction of the Peak Pressure on the Basis of Single Measurements

The peak, the trough, and the mean of diurnal variation curves that characterize the subjects studied are summarized in Table 1. The pressure variation was noted to be larger in the hypertensives than in the normotensive subjects. Least squares fitted curves to the data were obtained with the model $\underline{Yt} = \underline{M} + \underline{A} \cos (2\pi \underline{t} + \Phi)$, where $\underline{Yt}$ is the derived value at time $\underline{t}$, $\underline{M}$, $\underline{A}$, and Φ are the least squares derived coefficients, $\underline{M}$ = mesor, $\underline{A}$ = amplitude, and Φ = acrophase. Highly significant correlation was noted between the measured values and the values predicted on the basis of best fit cosine curve ($\underline{r} = +0.69$; $P < 0.05$). Characteristics of the rhythm are summarized in Table 2. A statistically significant correlation was demonstrated between the mesor ($\underline{M}$) and the amplitude ($\underline{A}$), indicating that the higher the mesor

Table 1. The peak, the trough, and the mean of diurnal variation (mm Hg)

	Highest IOP	Lowest IOP	Diurnal variation
Normal subjects	17.5 ± 0.28	11.1 ± 0.31	6.4 ± 0.20 (42)[a]
Ocular hypertensives	23.4 ± 0.35	15.0 ± 0.23	8.4 ± 0.30 (71)
Primary open-angle glaucoma patients	32.4 ± 1.12	19.1 ± 0.51	13.3 ± 0.83 (73)
Total	25.7 ± 0.59	15.8 ± 0.30	9.9 ± 0.39 (186)
Mean ± SEM.			

[a] The numbers in parentheses indicate the number of eyes

Table 2. Rhythms in IOP

	Mesor (mm Hg)	Amplitude (mm Hg)	Acrophase Ø (radian) Ø ref: 11:00 A.M.
Normal	14.4 ± 0.26	1.6 ± 0.10	0.16 ± 0.12 (42)[a]
Ocular hypertension	19.1 ± 0.27	2.2 ± 0.12	0.22 ± 0.07 (71)
Primary open--angle glaucoma	25.8 ± 0.83	3.7 ± 0.27	0.28 ± 0.07 (73)
Total subjects	20.8 ± 0.45	2.7 ± 0.13	0.23 ± 0.05 (186)

Rhythm detection: $\underline{P} < 0.05$ in each group; mean ± SEM.

[a] The numbers in parentheses indicate the number of eyes

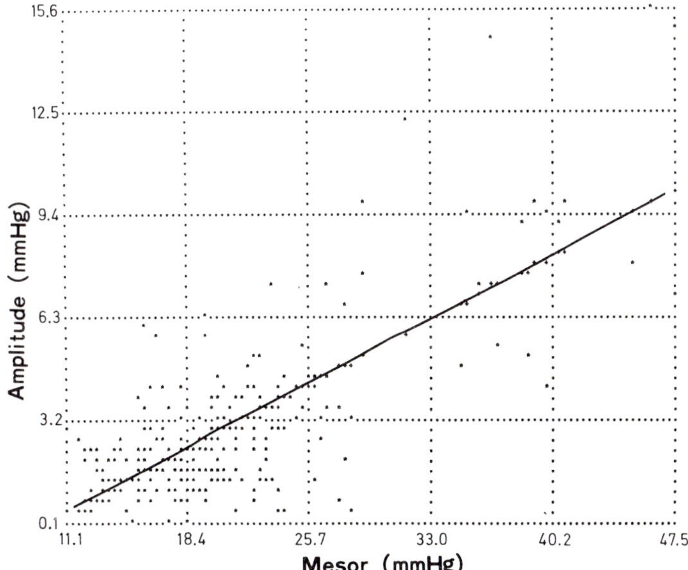

Fig.1. Correlation between mesor and amplitude

is the larger the amplitude is (Fig.1). This again is in keeping with the generally accepted concept that hypertensives have more marked pressure fluctuations than the normotensive subjects. The relationship between the peak pressure and the IOP measured every hour was analyzed on the basis of the first 200 determinations of diurnal curves. A highly significant correlation was noted between the IOP at 11:00 a.m. and the peak pressure ($\underline{r} = +0.98$; $P < 0.001$) and between the IOP at 12:00 noon and the peak pressure ($\underline{r} = +0.97$; $P < 0.001$). The relationship between IOP at 11:00 a.m. and the peak pressure is expressed as $\underline{Y} = 1.06\ \underline{X} + 0.96$, where $\underline{Y}$ = the peak pressure and $\underline{X}$ = IOP at 11:00 a.m. (Fig.2), and the relation-

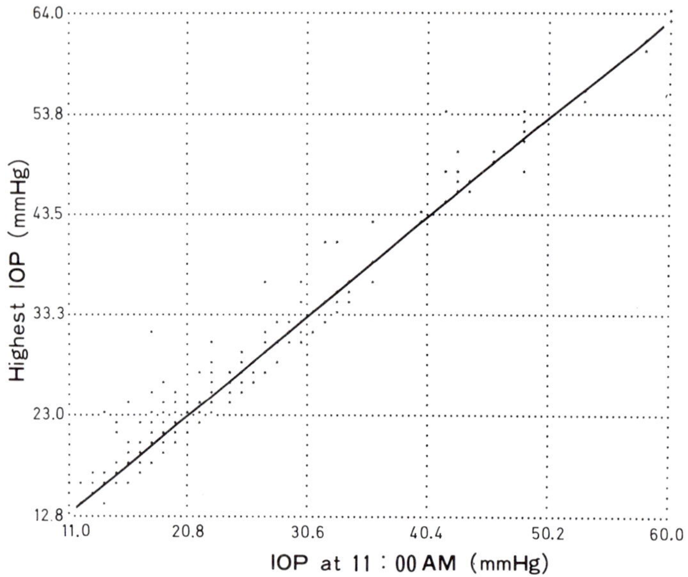

Fig.2. Relationship between IOP at 11:00 a.m. and the peak pressure

Table 3. The predicted and the measured peak on the basis of IOP at 11:00 A.M. (mm Hg)

Eye	IOP at 11:00 A.M.	Predicted peak (A)	Measured peak (B)	|A - B|
1	15	16.9	16	0.9
2	16	18.0	20	2.0
3	20	22.3	20	2.3
4	20	22.3	20	2.3
5	18	20.1	23	2.9
6	22	24.4	21	3.4
7	21	23.3	21	2.3
8	23	25.4	23	2.4
9	30	32.9	34	1.1
10	24	26.5	27	0.5
11	20	22.3	21	1.3
12	25	27.6	28	1.4
13	23	25.4	26	0.6
14	23	25.4	26	0.6
15	24	26.5	24	2.5
16	20	22.2	21	1.2
17	26	28.6	26	2.6
18	25	27.6	25	2.6
19	42	45.7	48	2.3
20	34	37.2	35	2.2
21	24	26.5	25	1.5
22	25	27.6	26	1.6
23	28	30.8	28	2.8
24	25	27.6	25	2.6
25	25	27.6	26	1.6
26	25	27.6	26	1.6
Mean	24.0	26.5	25.4	1.9

ship between IOP at 12:00 noon and the peak pressure is $\underline{Y} = 1.01\ \underline{X} + 2.24$, where $\underline{Y}$ = the peak pressure and $\underline{X}$ = IOP at 12:00 noon. The validity of the derived equations was tested on 26 eyes that later underwent hourly tonometry for 24 h. The IOP values at 11:00 a.m. and 12:00 noon were substitued for $\underline{X}$ in the equations, and the predicted values were compared with the actually determined peak values in each subject. The close agreement between the measured and the predicted peaks was demonstrated (Tables 3 and 4). The finding indicates strongly that tonometry late in the morning is useful in predicting the peak of the diurnal curve and that IOP at 11:00 a.m. is almost identical to the peak pressure. Since there is considerable evidence that the peaks of the IOP offer the greatest threat to the integrity of the visual function, a treatment program should take it into account to eliminate the peaks of pressure. Accordingly, the medical regimen for primary open-angle glaucoma should be designed in such a manner that the maximum hypotensive effect of the drug can be obtained late in the morning.

Period Preferable for the Evaluation of the Drug Effect

It has been known that the IOP in two eyes of an individual varies synchronously. For this reason, on evaluating the ocular hypotensive effect of the topically admin-

Table 4. The predicted and the measured peak on the basis of IOP at 12:00 A.M. (mm Hg)

Eye	IOP at 12:00 A.M.	Predicted peak (A)	Measured peak (B)	|A - B|
1	16	18.3	16	2.3
3	18	20.3	20	0.3
3	17	19.3	20	0.7
4	17	19.3	20	0.7
5	17	19.3	23	3.7
6	19	21.4	24	2.6
7	21	23.4	21	2.4
8	20	22.4	23	0.6
9	27	29.4	34	4.6
10	23	25.4	27	1.6
11	18	20.3	21	0.7
12	24	26.4	28	1.6
13	24	26.4	26	0.4
14	24	26.4	26	1.6
15	25	25.4	24	1.4
16	20	22.4	21	1.4
17	26	28.4	26	1.6
18	24	26.4	25	0.6
19	38	40.5	48	7.5
20	34	36.4	35	1.4
21	23	25.4	25	0.4
22	26	26.4	26	1.6
23	24	24.4	28	1.6
24	22	24.4	25	0.6
25	22	24.4	26	1.6
26	25	27.4	26	0.6
Mean	22.8	25.2	25.5	1.7

istered drug, one eye of individual subjects is treated and the fellow eye is kept untreated to serve as a control. Although the untreated fellow eye can serve as a control, it is desirable to choose a certain time period with the least pressure variation to determine the net drug effect exactly. Moreover, the knowledge of the time period with the least variation in a day is indispensable for the evaluation of the systemically administered hypotensive agent. The variations of IOP in different 6-h periods in a day were determined. It is apparent that the IOP varies least from 12:00 noon until 6:00 p.m. The magnitude of the variation during this particular period is more than 40% less as compared with that observed in the 8:00 a.m. to 2:00 p.m. period (Table 5).

Table 5. Variation of IOP during 6-h period in the daytime (mean ± SEM; n = 226)

Time	Variation of IOP[a]
7:00 A.M. - 1:00 P.M.	6.3 ± 0.31
8:00 A.M. - 2:00 P.M.	6.7 ± 0.25
9:00 A.M. - 3:00 P.M.	6.2 ± 0.29
10:00 A.M. - 4:00 P.M.	5.0 ± 0.17
11:00 A.M. - 5:00 P.M.	5.0 ± 0.17
12:00 A.M. - 6:00 P.M.	4.6 ± 0.15
1:00 P.M. - 7:00 P.M.	4.7 ± 0.19
2:00 P.M. - 8:00 P.M.	4.8 ± 0.19
3:00 P.M. - 9:00 P.M.	5.1 ± 0.22
4:00 P.M. - 10:00 P.M.	5.3 ± 0.25

[a] $$\frac{\sum_{n=1}^{226} (\text{highest IOP} - \text{lowest IOP})_n}{226}$$

Some Factors Related to the Magnitude of Diurnal Pressure Variation

Although the mechanisms generating the diurnal variation of the IOP remain to be elucidated, identification of the clinical factors that are somehow related to the magnitude of pressure variation is of clinical significance. The clinical factors including age, tonographic C value, the severity of field defects, and horizontal cup/disk ratio are evaluated in terms of their possible correlation with the magnitude of diurnal pressure variation. Statistically significant correlation was noted between tonographic C value and the magnitude of pressure variation in the test population as a whole ($r = -0.50$; $P < 0.001$, n = 226). In primary open-angle glaucoma patients, the age was noted to correlate well with the magnitude of pressure variation, and the correlation is expressed as $Y = -0.27\,X + 26.4$, where Y = magnitude of pressure variation and X = age in years ($r = -0.65$, $P < 0.001$, n = 87) (Fig.3). No significant relationship was demonstrated either between cup/disk ratio and the magnitude of pressure variation or between the severity of field changes and the magnitude of pressure variation. The correlation between C value and the magnitude of pressure variation is consistent with the previous reports postulating that the decreased and fixed outflow facility is responsible for the marked pressure variation in glaucoma, for it allows the pressure to be affected considerably by a small change in the aqueous formation. Little attention has been paid to the relationship of diurnal pressure variation to the biologic age. The finding that the magnitude of pressure variation is inversely proportional to the age in primary open-angle glaucoma patients has never been reported so far and warrants further investigation.

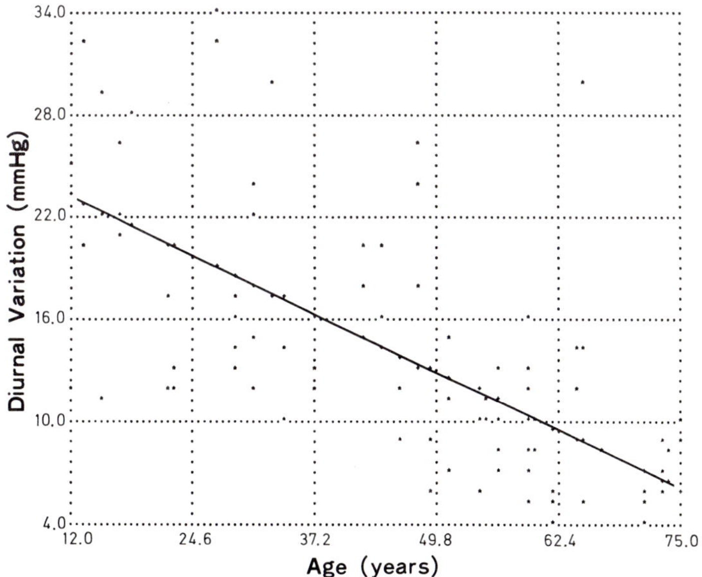

Fig.3. Correlation between age and magnitude of pressure variation in primary open-angle glaucoma patients.

Conclusion

The present study demonstrated that the detailed analysis of diurnal variation of the IOP can provide information useful in designing the medical regimen for the treatment of primary open-angle glaucoma and in evaluating the drug effects on the IOP;

1) The peak IOP correlated with the IOP measured at 11:00 a.m. and 12:00 a.m.; the correlation is statistically highly significant ($\underline{P} < 0.001$). The IOP at 11:00 or 12:00 a.m. enables one to predict the peak of IOP with accuracy.
2) IOP was noted to be most stable for 6 h from 12:00 to 6:00 p.m. during the day. This particular time interval may be most suitable for the evaluation of the immediate effect of the drug on the IOP.

3) The diurnal pressure variation was noted to be inversely proportional to the age in primary open-angle glaucoma patients and tonographically determined outflow facility in all the population studied.

References

(1) Drance, S.M.: The significance of the diurnal tension variations in normal and glaucomatous eyes. Arch. Ophthalmol. 64, 494 (1960)

(2) Erickson, L.A.: Twenty-four hourly variations in the inflow of the aqueous humor. Acta Ophthalmol. 36, 381 (1958)

(3) Henkind, P.; Leitman, M.; Weitzman, E.: The diurnal curve in man: new observations. Invest. Ophthalmol. 12, 705 (1973)

(4) Katavisto, M.: The diurnal variations of ocular tension in glaucoma. Acta Ophthalmol. [Suppl.] 78, 130 (1964)

(5) Kitazawa, Y.; Horie, T.: Diurnal variation of intraocular pressure in primary open-angle glaucoma. Am. J. Ophthalmol. 79, 557 (1975)

(6) Leydhecker, W.: The intraocular pressure: Clinical aspects. Ann. Ophthalmol. 8, 389 (1976)

(7) Newell, F.W.; Krill, A.E.: Diurnal tonography in normal and glaucomatous eyes. Trans. Am. Ophthalmol. Soc. 62, 349 (1964)

(8) Phelps, C.D.; Woolson, R.F.; Kolker, A.E.; Becker, B.: Diurnal variation in intraocular pressure. Am. J. Ophthalmol. 77, 367 (1974).

Discussion

LANGHAM: I noted that you took pressure readings every hour, and it is known that frequent applications of topical anesthetic will modify intraocular pressure. Can you exclude the possibility that anesthetic was partly responsible for your results, which appear to differ from those published by previous investigators?

KITAZAWA: There is a report in which diurnal curves were determined with a non contact tonometer without anesthesia, and the magnitude of variation was very similar to ours. So I think the effect of anesthesia has little to do with the magnitude of variation.

LICHTER: Is there evidence in the Japanese population that the diurnal variation in parameters other than intraocular pressure occur in the same time intervals those same variations in the Caucasian population? In other words, can we assume that the 11 a.m. high reading you found in the Japanese population also applies to the Caucasian population?

KITAZAWA: Although we know very little about the mechanisms that generate the spontaneous variation of intraocular pressure, I cannot see any reason why there should be a racial difference in the timing of peak pressure.

LEYDHECKER: The peak of intraocular pressure in most studies was found so far at 6:00 - 8:00 a.m. How do you explain this difference to your findings? SAMPAOLESI's results on the variation of intraocular pressure in normals were different and so were the results of Drance.

CALIXTO: One of our co-workers and myself, trying to simplify Sampaolesi's method of diurnal curve of pressure (DCP), have observed that its value is not changed when the 3:00 p.m. and 6:00 p.m. measurements are subtracted in the calculation. Thus, we found that statistically there were no differences with seven or five measurements for the diagnosis and for the clinical or surgical control of the disease. Possibly, the lower values obtained by Dr. KITAZAWA early in the morning are due to the time interval (5 min) between rising of the patient and the slit-lamp measurement.

KITAZAWA: We measured intraocular pressure on approximately 18 patients with a Perkins tonometer while patients were still in bed in the early morning (5:00 or

6:00 a.m.) and got very similar results. I cannot give you a good explanation of why our results contradict old concepts. The difference in the sleep-wake cycle of examinees might possibly be responsible for the discrepancy.

FRANÇOIS: I agree with Prof. LEYDHECKER and Prof. SAMPAOLESI. I also mostly found the highest intraocular pressure in the morning before 8:00 a.m., when the patient is still lying in bed and before he wakes up.

Response of the Intraocular Pressure to Various β-Blocking Agents

Günter K. Krieglstein

University Eye Hospital, Josef-Schneider-Straße 11,
D-8700 Würzburg, Germany (FRG)

β-Blocking compounds tend to be one of the cornerstones of the conservative management of chronic glaucoma. Because of the lack of interference with visual acuity, these drugs became more and more fashionable in glaucoma treatment. Basicly, β-blockers can be characterized pharmacologically by four criteria:

1) β-Blocking potency
2) β_1- or β_2-selectivity
3) Intrinsic sympathomimetic activity
4) Membrane-stabilizing effect.

Until now, we do not know to which criteria we should give preference in ophthalmology and which might be disadvantageous. The present paper reviews preliminary results on three β-blockers:

Timolol: non selective, no intrinsic sympathomimetic activity, no membrane-stabilizing effect
Bupranolol: non selective, no intrinsic activity, membrane-stabilizing effect
Metoprolol: β_1-selective, no intrinsic activity, no membrane-stabilizing effect.

Clinical Studies, Series I

The patients investigated in this series had been referred to the hospital because of insufficient intraocular pressure (IOP) control and glaucomatous field loss. In that respect they represented a selected group of progressed open-angle glaucomas. There was no previous history of β-blocking treatment in any of these patients. After discontinuation of glaucoma therapy for at least 48 h, a tension profile over 8 h was recorded without therapy. On the following day, the time-course of the IOP response to a single topical application of 0.5% timolol was recorded over 24 h. On the third and successive days, tension profiles were repeated under 0.5% timolol twice daily. Timolol treatment was discontinued when the mean of the tension profile exceeded 22 mm Hg.

Results

The mean time-course of the IOP of 39 glaucomatous eyes of series I is shown in Fig.1. There was an average IOP decrease of 13 mm Hg corresponding to 46% of the untreated pressure level. The individual effects scattered between 6 and 32 mm Hg

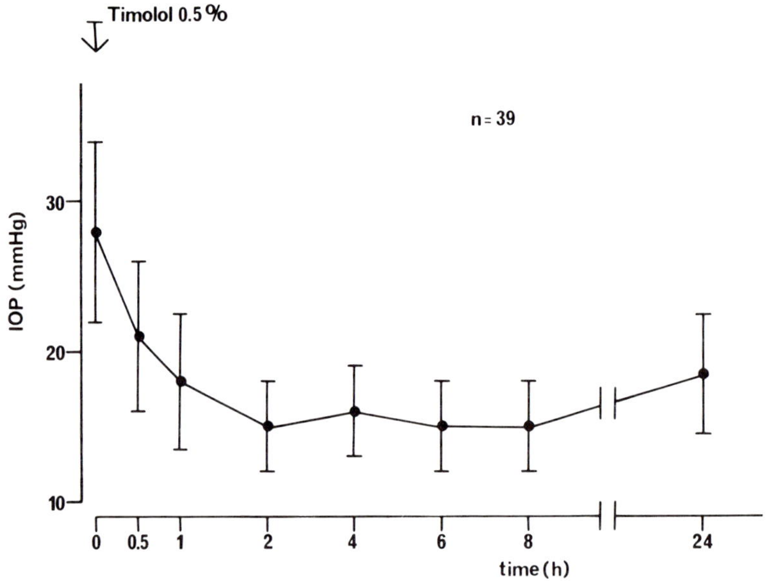

Fig.1. The mean time course of the IOP responses of 39 glaucomatous eyes to the local application of one drop of 0.5% timolol ophthalmic solution. The abscissa gives the time after treatment, the ordinate the intraocular pressure. Arithmetic means and the standard deviations of the means are presented.

(corresponding to 26% and 73% of the pressure level without therapy). However, 30 of 39 eyes of series I showed a gradual decrease of the IOP response within the first 3 days of repeated treatment with 0.5% timolol. The results were based on the means of tension profile of each day of treatment. Figure 2 compares the untreated pressure level with the mean initial response and the mean effect after repeated application of timolol 0.5% in these 30 eyes. The mean IOP on the 1st day of treatment was 17.3 mm Hg and on the 3rd day of treatment 23.6 mm Hg compared to 27.3 mm Hg without treatment. Eyes with fairly high IOP dominated that group.

Clinical Studies, Series II

Seven eyes of seven progressed open-angle glaucoma patients were studied in this series. After stopping antiglaucomatous therapy for 48h, bupranolol 1% twice daily was applied on the subsequent days. After development of subsensitivity against bupranolol therapy, tension profiles under timolol 0.5% twice daily were recorded.

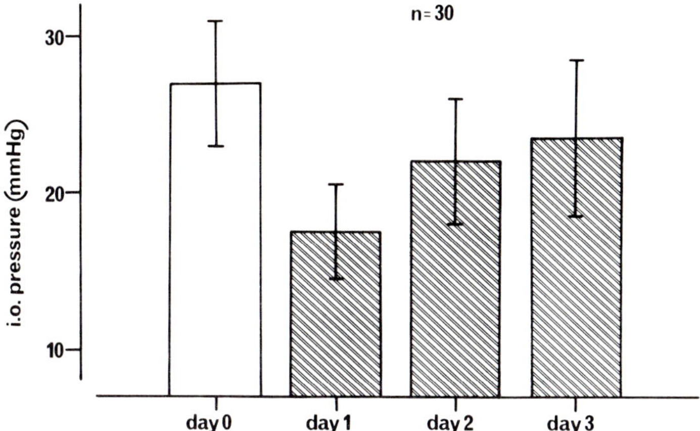

Fig.2. The IOP of 30 glaucomatous eyes within the first 3 days of treatment with 0.5% timolol. The first open column presents the untreated pressure levels based on the mean values of 30 day-tension curves without therapy. The columns with the diagonal lines present the treated pressure levels (mean values derived from profile tonometry under therapy; one application of 0.5% timolol on day 1, 0.5% timolol twice daily on days 2 and 3).

Results

The mean untreated pressure level in these seven patients was 38 mm Hg. On the 1st day of bupranolol treatment, the mean IOP was 21.4 mm Hg, an effect that is comparable to the initial response achieved with timolol therapy. On the 2nd to 4th day under bupranolol, the IOP averaged 25.7 mm Hg. Between the 3rd and 5th day of bupranolol treatment, the mean IOP returned to 30.1 mm Hg. The subsequent timolol treatment gave a mean IOP of 27.4 mm Hg. The comparative results of this series are shown in Fig.3. Timolol treatment after development of drug tolerance against the β-blocker bupranolol did not give the therapeutic response one would expect from the initial timolol therapy.

Clinical Studies, Series III

Twenty-two glaucomatous eyes of 11 open-angle glaucoma patients were studied in this series. After an interval of 48h without therapy, a tension profile was recorded over 8h after a single topical application of 0.1% timolol. To estimate the problem of drug tolerance to 0.1% timolol in this series of patients, tension profiles under 0.1% timolol twice daily were made on each subsequent day.

Results

The time-course of drug action after a single topical application of timolol 0.1% was not essentially different from that recorded with timolol 0.5% as shown in series I.

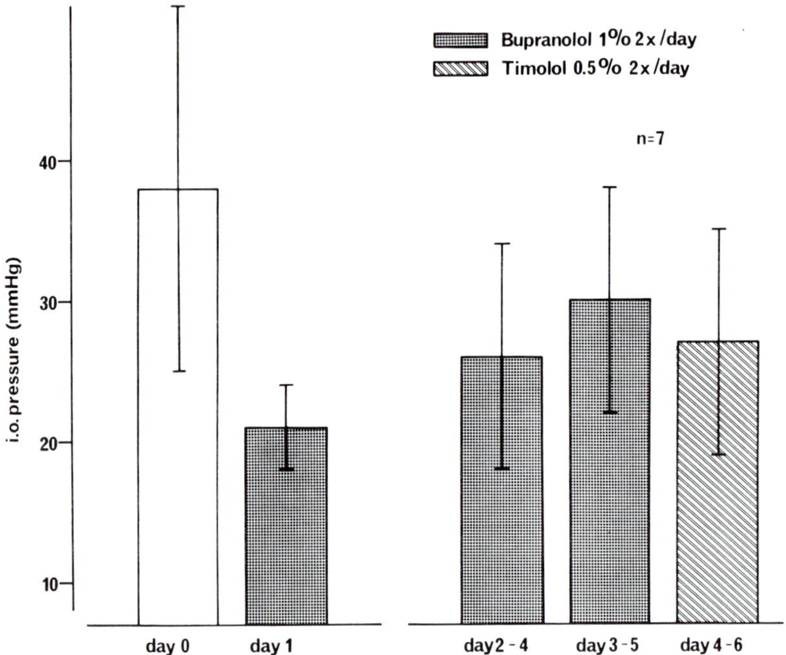

Fig.3. Comparison of bupranolol and timolol treatment in seven glaucomatous eyes. The first open column presents the untreated pressure level, the dotted columns present the pressure levels under bupranolol treatment over 3 - 5 days, the last column with diagonal lines indicates the IOP level under timolol treatment immediately following the bupranolol treatment (arithmetic means and standard deviations).

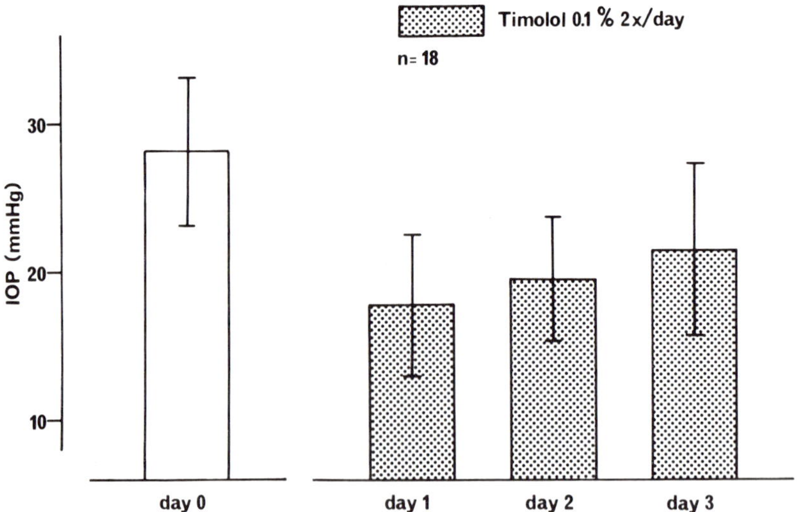

Fig.4. The mean IOP response of 18 glaucomatous eyes to 0.1% timolol twice daily on the first days of treatment. The open column gives the untreated pressure level, the dotted columns indicate the mean IOP on the first 3 days of treatment (mean ± SD).

The mean initial IOP decrease after drug administration in this series was 11.5 mm Hg (corresponding to 40% of the untreated pressure level). In 18 of 22 eyes, a careful day-by-day follow-up was possible. The average IOP in these eyes on the 1st day of treatment was 17.8 mm Hg compared to 21.7 mm Hg on the 3rd day of treatment. There was a partial loss of response to 0.1% timolol; however, it was less than observed with 0.5% timolol in series I. The mean IOP on the different days of treatment (based on tension profiles over 8 h) with 0.1% timolol is presented in Fig.4.

Clinical Studies, Series IV

Twenty-five hypertensive eyes of 13 patients (no glaucomatous cupping, no field loss) were investigated in this series. The untreated pressure levels were defined by tension profiles 48 h after discontinuation of therapy. The initial drug response to 0.25% timolol was established by profile tonometry in these eyes on the following day. Then the patients were put on 0.25% timolol twice daily. "To overcome patient error," the timolol eye drops were applied by the observer 12 h after the last drug application by the patient at each examination date. The time-course of timolol action was studied each time over 5 h (applanation pressure taken hourly). The average of three pressure readings seperated 1 h beginning 2 h after treatment was considered for the evaluation of the chronic response of 0.25% timolol. The observation period reported here is between 4 and 6 months.

Results

The initial therapeutic effects scattered between 6 and 20 mm Hg (10.8 mm Hg on the average, corresponding to 42% of the mean untreated pressure level). The average IOP response to 0.25% timolol treatment after 4 - 6 months was 6.5 mm Hg; this was a 25% decrease from the untreated pressure level. The gradual loss of response over a 6-month observation period is demonstrated in Fig.5. Starting with an initial mean response of 10.8 mm Hg, the average response after 1 month of treatment was 7.9 mm Hg, after 4 months 6.8 mm Hg, and after 6 months 5.6 mm Hg. In no eye did the tension return to pretreatment levels.

Clinical Studies, Series V

The β_1-selective β-blocker metoprolol had been investigated in four groups of open-angle glaucoma patients under blind conditions in this series. In a single-dose study, 0.1%, 0.5%, 1%, and 3% metoprolol eye drops were tested against placebo. Antiglaucomatous therapy was stopped 48 h prior to the test. The observer taking the pressures was not aware which eye had metoprolol treatment and which placebo solution.

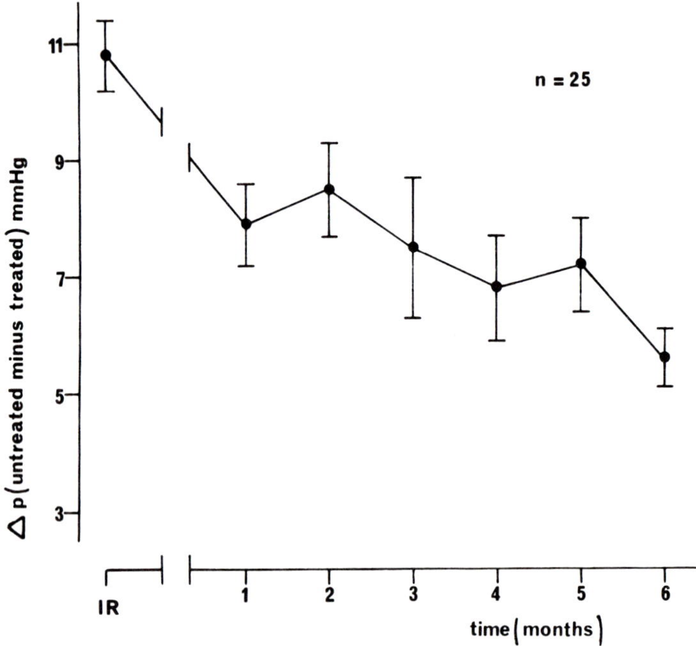

Fig.5. The IOP response to 0.25% timolol in 25 hypertensive eyes over 6 months treatment. The abscissa gives the duration of treatment, the ordinate the therapeutic effect (untreated minus treated pressure). IR, initial response (mean ± SD).

Results

Metoprolol 0.1% and 0.5% eye drops caused a small non significant IOP decrease after deduction of the placebo effect. Using metoprolol 1% and 3%, a marked IOP drop was noted within 2 h after treatment with a maximum of the effect after 4 h. Within 24 h the pressures in the treated eyes reached the pretreatment levels. The difference in the 1% and the 3% solution was statistically not significant. Both concentrations gave a mean IOP decrease of about 9 mm Hg, corresponding to 30% of the untreated pressure level. The dose-response relationship of metoprolol eye drops and IOP in glaucomatous eyes is presented in Fig.6.

In seven patients tested with the threshold concentration of 0.5% metoprolol, one drop 0.5% timolol was given 4 h after the metoprolol medication. A significant additive effect was noted. There was an additional response of timolol 0.5% of 8 mm Hg (metoprolol effect 5 mm Hg). The results of these combined treatments are presented in Fig.7.

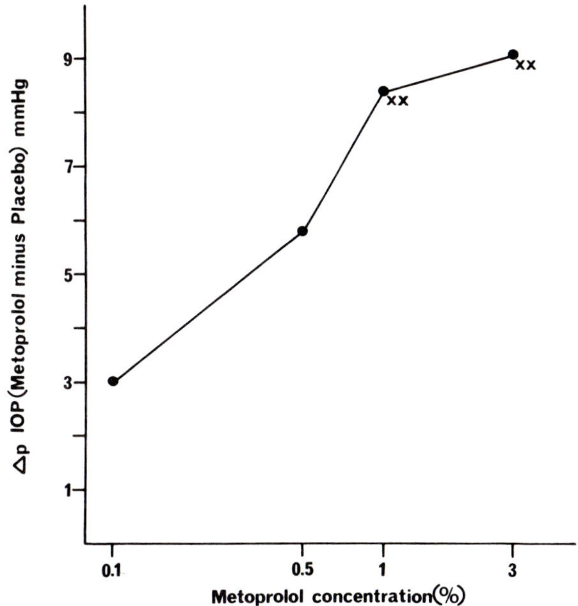

Fig.6. The dose-response curve of metoprolol ophthalmic solution and IOP. The abscissa shows the applied metoprolol concentrations, the ordinate the IOP responses (metoprolol response minus placebo response). Double crosses indicate statistical significance ($P < 0.01$).

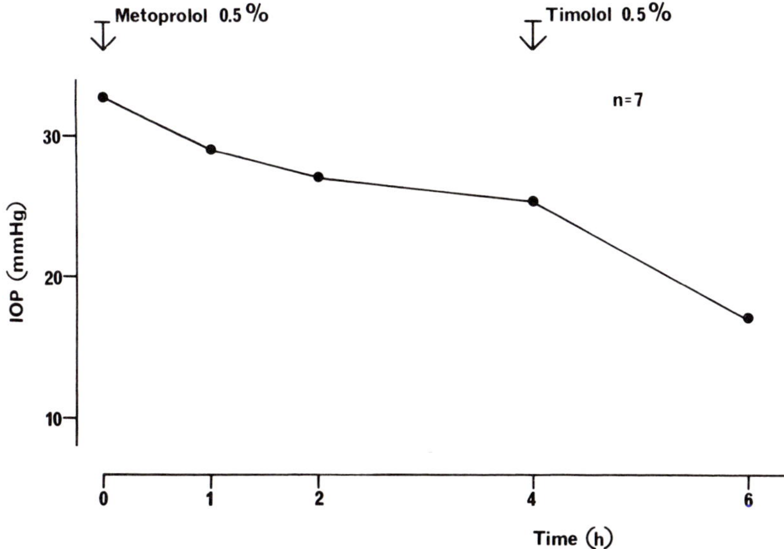

Fig.7. The additive effect of metoprolol and timolol eye drops on IOP. Four hours after a single topical application of metoprolol 0.5% to seven glaucomatous eyes of seven patients, timolol 0.5% drops were applied additionally. The abscissa gives the time after treatment, the ordinate the IOP (mean values).

Conclusions

1) The initial mean responses to timolol eye drops were as follows: 0.1% timolol 11.5 mm Hg, 0.25% timolol 10.8 mm Hg, and 0.5% timolol 13 mm Hg.
2) There was a gradual loss of response in the repeated administration of the drug.
3) The main part of drug adaptation happened in the 1st week of treatment; the magnitude of loss of response seems to be related to the untreated pressure level and the stage of the disease.
4) There is a large variety in the individual time-courses of drug adaptation with β-blockers (between days and several months).
5) Crossover studies revealed that development of drug tolerance to one β-blocker applies as well to an other.
6) The non selective β-blocker timolol appears to be more potent in reducing IOP than the β_1-selective metoprolol.
7) None of the tested β-blockers interfered with visual function, pupillary diameter, or systemic circuit.
8) IOP control by β-blocker therapy should include a careful follow-up in the 1st week of treatment especially in high IOPs because the initial overshooting response might be misleading.

Discussion

LEYDHECKER: The practitioner must be warned that he has to check patients under β-blockers still more carefully than those receiving pilocarpine. Adaptation is more frequent and much stronger with β-blockers: therefore, the chances are great that after 1 - 4 weeks the patient will have a higher pressure than on the 1st day of application of β-blockers. If the doctor does not check frequently enough, it could be possible that a patient with a quick adaptation to β-blockers has a high intraocular pressure soon after prescription, suffers a loss of visual fields, and the doctor discovers this deplorable development only at the next check after 2 or 3 months, when the field loss is irreversible. However, β-blockers are very useful in preparing a patient for surgery, especially in a case of cataract extraction combined with glaucoma. There is no better means to have a low pressure at the time of surgery than when β-blockers are given for 4 h prior to surgery. However, this will work only if the patient has not been previously treated with these drugs.

LEE: Timolol is useful alternative agent in the management of patients who are either allergic or hypersensitive to topical epinephrine and/or pilocarpine. Eleven primary open-angle glaucoma patients with allergic and/or hypersensitive reaction to topical epinephrine and/or pilocarpine tolerated timolol well up to 3 - 6 months in the follow-up period. The therapeutic effect is at least equal to epinephrine.

DRANCE: In answer to Prof. LEYDHECKER's question, we have found on single instillation of pilocarpine that 4% and 8% do not have a greater pressure reduction than 2% but the duration is much longer. It should be remembered that all drugs reduce pressure best immediately after they are started and the effect then gradually wears off. This is not only a function of the β-adrenergic agonists and antagonists.

LEYDHECKER: I do not agree with Dr. DRANCE. The very slow wearing of the pilocarpine effect usually takes months or years. It is caused by a progress of the disease, presumably an increase in outflow resistance. This is something fundamentally different from the quick adaptation to β-blockers that usually occurs within 3 days.

PODOS: Reduced response to a drug is not only characteristic of timolol but of the other drugs in use. Despite that adaptation, timolol has a better effect than epinephrine or pilocarpine in comparative studies. Drs. MOSS, RITCH, KOHN, and I have carried out a double-masked crossover study comparing timolol and epinephrine in the same 36 patients. More patients were controlled with timolol than epinephrine, and timolol produced a significantly greater drop in the intraocular pressure than epinephrine in this study up to 6 weeks after initiating therapy.

FRANÇOIS: May I ask Dr. KRIEGLSTEIN if with timolol he obtained in some cases a pressure reduction of more than 20 mm Hg. I never found a reduction of more than 15 - 20 mm Hg. For those who have difficulties in obtaining timolol, I will give you a simple prescription. One takes two tablets of blocadren, which is commercially available and which is timolol used orally for angina pectoris. These two tablets are mixed with 3 ml of distilled water and then filtered. These 3 ml are mixed with another 3 ml of distilled water and again filtered. You thus obtain a solution of timolol at 0.5%.

KRIEGLSTEIN: The maximum effects after starting β-blocker therapy we found were up to 32 mm Hg. However, these effects corresponding 70% of the untreated pressure level in these cases could be maintained just for 2 or 3 days, then a marked decrease in the initial response occurred.

GREVE: In our department, Dr. ROS studied atenolol, metropotol, and recently timolol. We found adaptation both to atenolol (as did PHILLIPS) and to metropolol (as did KRIEGLSTEIN). It is for the first time now that we hear that timolol also shows adaptation, although this has not yet been published.
I should like to ask your attention for another very potent drug or drug combination. Dr. HOYNG from our department will give a report on guanethidine (3%) and epinephrine (0.5%) in Kyoto (1) Guanethidine creates a supersensitivity to epinephrine causing a long-term reduction of intraocular pressure that is as much as 35% - 40%. This means that it is more potent than any of the local β-blocking drugs.
The disadvantages of the guanethidine-epinephrine combination are the same as that of epinephrine. Our main problem has been the development of red-eye syndrome 3 h after application of the drop. Guanethidine has been found very useful in the management of glaucoma patients, either alone or in combination with pilocarpine and diamox.

ZIMMERMAN: This was a fine summary of multiple clinical studies with several of the β-blockers. I would only like to comment on the "loss of effect" of the β-blockers. In addition to your work, there is mounting evidence that strongly suggest that some of the β-blockers suffer from true tachyphylaxis, that is, the loss of the entire effect after a short time of continued use of the drug. The β-blocker that I am most familiar with is timolol, and I was pleased to see that your results concerning this drug are quite similar to mine. Specifically, concerning the loss of effect of timolol, you have pointed out a finding that I have only recently become aware of from my own studies. Once again, we have similar results in that there is waning of the initial ocular hypotensive effect within the first few weeks or months of therapy. In my patients, I find the initial pressure drop to be around 40%. After several weeks, this response decreases to approximately 30%, and as you have also found this seems to be the effect that lasts. In over 50 patients followed for 1 year, the above-described pressure response seems clear, and the 30% decrease in IOP does not seem to further deteriorate. Again, I congratulate you on your fine work.

Principles and Selection of Surgical Methods in Primary Glaucoma

H. Harms

University Eye Hospital, Schleichstraße 12, D-7400 Tübingen, Germany (FRG)

In the last 3 decades, the conditions for surgical interventions in glaucoma have changed. We have a better knowledge of the pathogenesis of primary glaucoma, and improvements in microsurgery enable us to develop new surgical methods.

Soon the report on a study done under the auspices of the German Ophthalmologic Society (DOG) will be published. In a prospective study in co-operation with 32 eye departments, success and risk of different procedures in open-angle glaucoma were investigated. Conventional fistulizing procedures, the fistulizing operations with a scleral cover and the trabeculotomy, could be compared.

The limits for the "normal level" of intraocular pressure (IOP) were assumed to be between 10 - 21 mm Hg. The mean of the diurnal pressure was taken from five measurements between 8:00 a.m. and 6:00 p.m. There is a total number of 519 operated cases with a follow-up period of 1 year. For the evaluation of the differences, their significances had to be calculated. Due to the limited number of follow-up cases, our evaluation may be regarded as general advice only.

Pathogenesis of Elevation of the IOP

The pathologic elevation of the IOP in primary glaucoma mainly caused by an obstruction of the outflow of aqueous humor. The aim of the surgical procedure is to restore a sufficient outflow of aqueous humor. The more exact the localization of the obstruction of the outflow, the more precise the necessary operation can be performed in each individual case.

Pupillary block and angle closure can be easily recognized. In open-angle glaucomas, the increased outflow resistance is located in the inner wall of Schlemm's canal or in its outer wall or in both places. It has become obvious that in most cases the localization is found in the trabecular meshwork. We also may conclude this from the positive results after trabeculotomy. However, it is also observed after trabeculotomy that despite a clear rupture of the trabecular meshwork the IOP is not normalized, or in single cases not even influenced at all. In those cases the outflow resistance must at last be partially located in the outer wall. For an optimal performance of a surgical intervention in each single case, we should be able to determine the exact location of the outflow resistance beforehand.

Principles and Mechanisms of Action in the Different Glaucoma Operations

There are three surgical principles to lower the IOP:

1) To restore the physiologic outflow facilities sufficiently
2) To provide new ways of outflow
3) To restrict the production of aqueous humor.

Iridectomy, goniotomy, and trabeculotomy belong to the first group. The mechanism of action of the iridectomy is quite evident and unquestioned. Goniotomy after BARKAN is basically a trabeculotomy ab interno. There is no discussion about its mechanism of action, which opens the outflow possibility via Schlemm's canal. In the case of trabeculotomy ab externo (BURIAN, R. SMITH), the same mechanism shall be effective. Therefore, after rupture of the trabecular meshwork, the scleral lamella is sutured watertight over the outer opening of Schlemm's canal to avoid an additional outflow of aqueous humor under the conjunctiva. A filtering bleb, of course, can develop if the suture is not closed sufficiently. Some authors, however, assume that in those cases of trabeculotomy without filtering bleb pressure decrease takes place by microfiltration under the conjunctiva. Histologic proof of this opinion is not known to us. The clinical experience, however, argues against it. When comparing the mean pressure, it shows that 1 year after operation the pressure decrease after trabeculotomy is not as high as with all other fistulizing operations (Table 1). There is no difference in the height of the pressure between those cases <u>with</u> and those <u>without</u> filtering bleb (Table 2). This makes it doubtful that the thickening of the conjunctiva after trabeculotomy is a "filtering bleb." In my opinion, we may assume that trabeculotomy belongs to those surgical interventions restoring the normal outflow of aqueous humor.

To the second group, i.e., provision of new ways of outflow, all fistulizing procedures have to be counted, including those with additional scleral cover. Its mechanism can be proved by filling the anterior chamber with fluoresceinate and observing the outflow of aqueous humor. Recently, BENEDIKT (1) carried out detailed investigations on the outflow of aqueous humor, especially after trabeculectomy. He found that the outflow occurs mainly via a subconjunctival exit of aqueous humor connected to lymphatic vessels or by direct transport of aqueous humor through newly formed water veins and lymphatic vessels from the operating field.

The third principle in the surgical glaucoma treatment of glaucoma is the partial coagulation of the ciliary body to restrict the production of aqueous humor, which

Table 1.

Surgical technique	n	Mean intraocular pressure (mm Hg) Preoperative	Postoperative
Scheie	59	31.6	13.6
Iridencleisis	61	34.0	15.2
Elliot	54	28.2	13.9
Scheie with scleral cover	33	32.7	15.8
Elliot with scleral cover	74	29.4	14.4
Trabeculotomy	62	30.5	19.5
$\sum$	343	30.9	15.4

Table 2.

1 year after trabeculotomy	n	Arithmetic mean of intraocular pressure	Filtering bleb 1 year after trabeculotomy	Mean intraocular pressure (mm Hg) ≤ 21	21,1 - 24	> 24
With filtering bleb	15	18.73 mm Hg	Yes	11	3	1
Without filtering bleb	62	18.66 mm Hg	No	44	13	5

should be adapted to the impaired outflow facility. This procedure causes a diffuse trauma of the sclera by cryo- or diathermy coagulation. The varying thickness of the sclera (0.3 - 1.3 mm) makes it impossible to estimate how deep and to what extent the diathermy has changed the ciliary body. From our clinical experience, we know that the coagulation of the ciliary body often only causes a temporary pressure decrease. However, in quite a remarkable percent of the cases a lasting pressure decrease could be observed. A complication that is not rare - mostly after repeated cyclodiathermy - is hypotony with phtisis bulbi. The mechanism of action of the pressure lowering in this procedure is not yet understood sufficiently.

Pressure-Lowering Effect of Different Glaucoma Operations

In general, the advantage of a glaucoma operation is judged from its effect on lowering the IOP. This effect is considered as being too low if the pressure still ranges above the upper limit of the normal level. Less consideration, however, is given to a pressure below the normal level.

Table 1 shows that after SCHEIE's and ELLIOT's operation the average pressure is found to be to 2 - 3 mm below the mean pressure, after trabeculotomy, however,

3 - 4 mm above the normal pressure. The different effects of the pressure decrease of the various methods become more evident when subdividing the pressure values into three groups (Table 3). The conventional fistulizing operations show postoperatively in a great percent a pressure below the normal range, whereas the trabeculotomy shows a great percent pressure values above the normal range. Splitting the pressure values into six groups for each surgical method (Table 4), we gain the additional information that the higher pressure values after trabeculotomy still range within the 3-σ limit of the normal mean pressure.

Table 3.

Surgical technique	n	(%)	Postoperative mean intraocular pressure < 10.0		10.0 - 21.0		> 21	
FO[a] (conventional)	203	(100)	42	(21)	142	(70)	19	(9)
FO with scleral cover	108	(100)	7	(7)	92	(85)	9	(8)
Trabeculotomy	77	(100)	1	(1)	54	(70)	22	(29)

[a] FO, filtering operation

Table 4.

Surgical technique	Postoperative mean intraocular pressure (mm Hg) frequency distribution (percent) n	< 10.0	10.0 - 13.0	13.1 - 19.0	19.1 - 21	21.1 - 24	> 24
Scheie	75	21	23	47	5	1	3
Iridencleisis	74	19	22	38	11	1	9
Elliot	54	22	30	28	6	7	7
Scheie with scleral cover	33	9	22	48	3	12	6
Elliot with scleral cover	75	5	24	64	3	4	-
Trabeculotomy	77	1	2	47	21	21	8

Risks of the Different Glaucoma Operations

The differences in the operating risk are demonstrated in the postoperative deterioration of the visual acuity (Table 5). This example is chosen because the operation is performed with the aim of preserving the visual acuity. In Table 6, the operating methods are classified according to the frequency of deterioration and the significance, as far as existent. We cannot go into details, but we would like to emphasize that significant differences in the risks exist.

Table 5.

Decrease of visual acuity [ratio 1 year postop. over preop.]									
Surgical technique	n	No < 0.06		Small 0.06 - 0.25		Considerable 0.26 - 0.55		Large > 0.55	
Scheie	95	34	(36)	27	(28)	23	(24)	11	(12)
Iridencleisis	103	45	(44)	24	(23)	18	(17)	16	(16)
Elliot	63	27	(43)	17	(27)	14	(22)	5	(8)
Scheie with scleral cover	38	28	(73)	4	(11)	2	(5)	4	(11)
Elliot with scleral cover	92	49	(53)	25	(27)	8	(9)	10	(11)
Trabeculotomy	128	80	(62)	20	(16)	22	(17)	6	(5)
$\sum$	519	263	(51)	117	(22)	87	(17)	52	(10)

Table 6. Significant frequency differences of the decrease of visual acuity 1 year after different surgical techniques [see Table 5]

> 0.06 small + considerable + large				> 0.25 considerable + large				> 0.55 large			
Scheie	wsc[a]	27%		Scheie	wsc	16%		TT		5%	
TT[b]		38%		Elliot	wsc	20%		Elliot		8%	
Elliot	wsc	47%	s s	TT		22%		Elliot	wsc	11%	
JCL[c]		56%	s s	Elliot		30%		Scheie	wsc	11%	
Elliot		57%	s s	JCL		33%	s s	Scheie		12%	
Scheie		64%	s s s	Scheie		36%	s s s	JCL		16%	s

[a] wsc - with scleral cover
[b] TT - trabeculotomy
[c] JCL - iridencleisis

Suggestions for the Improvement of Operative Glaucoma Treatment

Considering everything being said about the mechanism of action of the different surgical interventions, about its effect and its risk, we must admit that we still stand on an unsteady ground with regard to the decision for a certain operative procedure. I believe, however, that by means of prospective research our surgical therapy can be improved. We would like to discuss the following requirements:

1) The exact localization of the increased resistance should be possible preoperatively. An interesting approach has been carried out by BENEDIKT to study the

outflow channels by means of fluorescein filling of the anterior chamber pre- and postoperatively. In this context, the suggestion of GROTE to fill Schlemm's canal with fluorescein would possibly allow us to differentiate the outflow resistance in the trabecular meshwork and the outer wall.

2) The mechanism of action of the three operating principles have to be analyzed more precisely by the study of the postoperative outflow conditions. Mixing up of different principles in one method should therefore be avoided.

3) The operating methods have to be changed in a way that the traumatization of the eye is reduced to a minimum. Such suggestions are the "transcorneal access to the chamber angle" (5) and the "direct cauterisation of the ciliary body" (4).

4) The methods for restriction of the production of the aqueous humor should be investigated more exactly in animal experiments.

5) Careful clinical observations on the pressure-decreasing effect and the complications of the different glaucoma operations have to be continued.

It is suggested that small study groups for certain limited research tasks be established based on the International Glaucoma Club.

References

(1) Benedikt, O.: Die Darstellung des Kammerwasserabflußes normaler und glaukomkranker menschlicher Augen durch Füllung der Vorderkammer mit Fluorescein. Albrecht von Graefes Arch. Klin. Ophthalmol. 199, 45-67 (1976)

(2) Goldmann, H.; Lotmar, W.: Rapid detection of changes in the optic disc: Stereo-Chronoscopy. Albrecht von Graefes Arch. Klin. Ophthalmol. 202, 87-99 (1977)

(3) Grote, P.: Untersuchungen zur Indikationsstellung der Trabekulotomie bei Glaukoma simplex. Zur Darstellung der Kammerwasserabflußwege mit Fluorescein. (in press (1978)

(4) Grote, P.; Harms, H.: Erste Ergebnisse der direkten Ziliarkörperkauterisation (DZK). Ber. dtsch. ophthalmol. Ges. 74, 661-665 (1977)

(5) Harms, H.: Transcornealer Zugang zum Kammerwinkel. Ber. Dtsch. Ophthalmol. Ges. 74, [Suppl.] 647-650 (1977).

Discussion

FRANÇOIS: I agree that one has less often a cataract after trabeculectomy than after another filtering operations, although the percent after trabeculectomy is also rather high. On the other hand, we have to differentiate between cortical cataract and nuclear cataract. Cortical opacities are, I think, not due to the operation but to age, while nuclear cataract may be due to the operation itself.

DRANCE: I would like to comment on cataract formation after operation. We reported on a 3-year follow-up of trabeculectomy and Scheie's procedure in consecutive patients operated by one surgeon. There was a significantly smaller incidence of cataracts after the trabeculectomy, probably because of the flap and the freedom of anterior chamber loss.

LEYDHECKER: Prof. HARMS has to be congratulated on his attempt to analyze the results of surgery. The great difficulty in any such study is that one has to combine results from surgeons of different quality. This also applies to my earlier report on the late results of surgery from the Bonn University Eye Hospital, in which different surgeons took part. The surgical techniques at Bonn were from the same school. However, in the study at Tübingen, different surgical schools and the work of surgeons with extremely different surgical ability and technique have been combined. I am not sure that many general conclusions can be drawn from an inhomogeneous material. Specifically, cataract development was found in the old age group only, but is was not stated how often cataract occurred in that age group without surgery. One certainly cannot generalize that iridencleisis causes cataract at such and such a percent, since the Tübingen material contained only the older method of Holth by knife incision and the incarceration of two iris pillars. With my own method of peripheral iridencleisis, which was not included in the Tübingen study, I have a few patients in whom one eye was treated with this peripheral iridencleisis, while the other eye remained unter treatment by miotics. After 1 year, the frequency of increase in lens opacities was less in the operated eyes than in the eyes with medical treatment. My interpretation is that in these eyes the lens opacities followed the pattern of development that they would have shown without any treatment or surgery and that, in these cases, iridencleisis did not accelerate cataract development. The reason is, I suppose, that the anterior chamber is never lost during the operation with peripheral iridencleisis. Therefore, the lens is never deprived of its nourishing aqueous humor. Some clinically interesting questions were insufficiently registered in the Tübingen study. For example, the question of whether steroids can prevent cicatrization cannot be answered from the study, because in the questionnaire it was only asked whether a subconjunctival injection at the end of the operation was done or not, while further postoperative treatment with steroids was not registered. It was also not registered whether the pupil was kept dilated or not during the postoperative days. My own report on late results of glaucoma surgery has been published in the Tutzing Symposion (1). I do not want to go into the details of this study, but I would just like to point out that the most important cause for a lens deterioration was the age of the patient.

Reference

(1) Leydhecker, W. (ed.): Glaucoma Symposion. Tutzing Castle, 1966. Basel: Karger 1967.

KRASNOV: For a number of years, I worked with the so-called sinusotomy (externalization of Schlemm's canal) by which the canal lumen is opened from outside. I am happy to hear today that Prof. HARMS admits the possibility of the existence of the obstacle to aqueous outflow at the outer wall of Schlemm's canal. This was also substantiated recently by works of Sawada and Langham et al. But I want to call your attention to another fact. As I mentioned, we have worked with sinusotomy. We have also worked with Harms' trabeculotomy and found it to be very elegant and effective. Nowadays, we have extensive experience with the so-called trabeculectomy of Cairns. It is interesting that all of these procedures, at least in our hands, gave approximately the same rate of success as far as their hypotensive action are concerned. I wonder if Prof. HARMS would like to comment on it. In my opinion, it probably has something to do with the so-called Schlemm's canal collapse (Nesterov et al.). All of the above procedures may influence this condition strongly.

SHAFFER: Decreased visual acuity following surgery is frequently caused by cataract formation. It is true that there is a 10% increase in cataracts in normal unoperated cases over the age of 70 years. This must be subtracted from postoperative cataract statistics. We agree that cataract production is certainly greater after any operation. Formation is less in trabeculectomy and in trabeculotomy because the postoperative inflammation is less and the pressure somewhat higher than in conventional filtering procedures. Even following iridectomy as a prophylactive procedure, there is an increase in cataract formation over a 10-year period.

HETHERINGTON: In a limited group of patients evaluated, we found a very low success rate in older patients (40 and over) and a much higher success level in the younger age group especially patients under 20 years of age.
Dr. HARMS, did you not study results in younger patients? I would like to ask Dr. KRASNOV how it was possible that - as he said - 60% of patients were able to avoid surgery. For how long was this possible?

KRASNOV: For 5 years at the longest. However, it is necessary to perform four laser treatments in a year.

SIVA REDDY: In cases of primary congenital glaucoma, in my experience in India, goniotomy is a safe surgical method. It has good results. In a few cases, trabeculotomy and trabeculectomy were performed with good results. When both these operations failed, how do you manage these cases, Prof. HARMS?

KITAZAWA: It is well-known that goniotomy, which is essentially "trabeculotomy ab interno," does not work in adult primary open-angle glaucoma. I wonder why trabeculotomy ab externo works and the ab interno procedure does not.

LEE: 1) Our clinical experience as well as the work of Drs. SCHAFFER and HETHERINGTON are in agreement with Prof. HARMS' data that the pressure-lowering effect is greater with the Elliot trephine than with other types of filtering procedures.
2) Our experience showed that trabeculotomy is not very effective in pressure reduction in old patients.
3) With our modified trabeculectomy procedure, we can achieve a greater pressure reduction effect than with standard trabeculectomy. In a 3 - 5-year postoperative follow-up study, we found that pressure below 15 mm Hg occurred in 65% - 70%, with an overall successful result of 84%. Visual function decreased at a rate of about 1% - 1.5% per year. Cataract occurred in 3 of the 32 eyes 3 - 5 years after the operation.

KRIEGLSTEIN: It is important to watch the incidence of cataract formation in the operated eye against the untreated eye intra individually. We feel that the intra individual comparison does not give the overall answer but might be superior to comparing operated eyes in different subjects.

HERSCHLER: We have been taught by Dr. SHAFFER that "it is not the quality of the wound, but the quality of the wounded." Success rates of filtering surgery are most likely more dependent upon case selection than upon the type of operation performed. My preliminary work with aqueous humor inhibition of conjunctival fibroblasts in tissue culture shows a significant correlation between aqueous behavior and the chances for surgical success.

HARMS (closing remarks): You will have noticed that it was not my intention to demonstrate the advantages and disadvantages of certain operations. I believe that in some respect the material from the study of the German Ophthalmologic Society is not large enough and in any case it is not yet finally evaluated. We hope that in a later stage we can carefully consider the different operation methods. Today, I only wanted to show that there are differences between the methods. LEE and KTASAMA have referred to a different pressure lowering in the different procedures. In conformity with us, SHAFFER found that opacities of the lens occur after any operation, however, to a different extent. The influence of age with regard to the extent of the pressure lowering, as found by HETHERINGTON and LEE, could not be gathered from our material, which, in my opinion is not very suitable for such an evaluation because the percent of young operated patients is very low. KRASNOV has found the same rate of pressure lowering after sinusotomy, trabeculotomy, and trabeculectomy and ask, if this might be caused by a collapse of Schlemm's canal. I already emphatically pointed out that in my opinion, the investigation of the mechanism of action of the different methods should be one of our most important tasks. Since a different extent of pressure lowering is also shown in the different methods, it is obvious to believe in a different mechanism of action. Therefore, in this respect, the recent investigations of BENEDIKT seem to me of special importance. BENEDIKT had already reported in detail about the outflow of the aqueous humour after trabeculectomy and other filtering operations. However, recently he also investigated some patients with the same procedure after trabeculotomy. He was so kind to make some slides available to me for this discussion. In the example shown, no outflow through an aqueous vein can be seen in the photograph made before the operation, but according to the explanations of BENEDIKT a slight admixture of aqueous humour must have been visible by slit-lamp observation. The two following photographs were made some weeks after trabeculotomy. Now you can see that the fluorescinated aqueous humour flows out via a typical aqueous vein. According to BENEDIKT, this finding basically differs from all his experiences with fistulizing operations including trabeculectomy [CAIRNS.]

Therefore, we must assume that in this case a different mechanism of action has taken place, i.e., a reopening of the outflow facilities through the aqueous veins after rupture of the trabecular meshwork. BENEDIKT will surely report about his results so that I do not want to give further explanations at this time.

Without doubt, we do not know enough about the mechanism of action and the complications of our different surgical methods. I absolutely agree with Herschler that the individual reaction on the surgical trauma might also be of great importance for the success of the intervention. Therefore, I think it is necessary to change the methods in such a way that the traumatization of the eye is reduced to a minimum. In our statistical material originating from 32 different eye departments, this individually different reaction to surgery cannot explain the differences that we saw between the methods.

It is known to me that at present one tries - if possible - to avoid a surgical intervention in glaucoma treatment. However, I am convinced that we cannot do without sursurgical treatment. If this is correct, it is necessary to make a critical comparison of the operations and reconsider the indication for a certain procedure.

Laser Treatment in Glaucoma

M.M. Krasnov

Director State Institute of Ophthalmology, 5 Pogodinskaja st.,
Moscow 119435, USSR

Several possible uses of laser for glaucoma treatment have currently been introduced, its assessment ranging from promising to reliable. The main fields of clinical application are:

1) Laser iridectomy for narrow-angle glaucoma
2) Laser iridectomy as a prophylactic measure against an acute attack of the narrow-angle glaucoma on a fellow eye
3) Laser trabeculopuncture for the "simple" ("wide-angle") glaucoma.

Potentialities of some other laser procedures deserve closer scientific study: laser gonioplasty (tangential coagulation of the iris as termed by HAGER), laser goniospasis, and posterior cyclocoagulation. All the above procedures have been tried in the author's clinical practice.

Different types of laser proved more or less suitable for each particular method of treatment. The action of the commonly used lasers (such as, for instance, argon gas or long-pulsed ruby) is primarily thermal. This accounts for some undesirable side-effects due to the tissue burn.

A considerable part of the effect produced by the Q-switched lasers can be termed "mechanical" (although, actually, this is a combination of many effects). A combined use of different lasers can be very beneficial, for instance, in iridectomy.

A laser iridotomy can fairly often be produced with conventional (long-pulsed ruby or argon gas) lasers (3). The chances of success depend considerably on the technical skill of the operator. Using an argon gas laser (coherent radiation, model 800), it was possible to make a through- and-through hole in the iris in about 78% of patients with narrow-angle glaucoma. Multiple (up to 200 and more) short pulses of low energy were used and the procedure was quite safe and non-traumatic.

More than 300 laser iridectomies have so far been performed in our clinical practice. On the whole, the problem of laser iridectomy seems to be scientifically solved.

Its hypotensive result (and, consequently, its clinical value) may, however, be somewhat different from that following a surgical iridectomy because the external filtration is absent. Being practically harmless, the laser iridectomy must be performed as early as possible to avoid the formation of peripheral goniosynechias.

The "prophylactic" laser iridectomy on the fellow eye after an acute attack of narrow-angle glaucoma seems to be of unquestionable clinical value. The procedure of laser gonioplasty ("tangential coagulation of the iris" as termed by HAGER (1)) can also be quite helpful, but usually for temporary relief or as a sort of pretreatment. Thirty to fifty laser coagulations are delivered to the root of the iris, immediately causing some shrinkage of the tissue, which usually recedes from the angle.

It has been shown by several authors that a laser goniopuncture can successfully be carried out with the use of conventional coagulating lasers (4). The thermal burn to the angle structures is followed by an inflammatory response. As a result, the trabecular meshwork is replaced by a connective tissue scar. That was the fundamental starting point in our work with Q-switched lasers. Their action is mainly mechanical (disruptive), and hence, it was more or less conveniently labeled a "cool" laser. So far the method has been tried on the eyes of 189 patients. All of them faced glaucoma surgery and the Q-switched laser goniopuncture was for them the last chance to avoid it. The clinical effectiveness of the method is best illustrated by the fact that in two-thirds of these cases surgical treatment was avoided. To date, some of these patients have been followed up for 5 years. Improvement in out flow facility was a characteristic finding. The procedure can (and often should) be used repeatedly on the same eye. It seems that it can successfully limit the use of surgery in open-angle glaucoma.

A new method of the so-called laser goniospasis has been investigated during the last 2 years. It was termed after Cairn's surgical procedure because its aim is basically the same. About 30 laser coagulations are placed to the anterior part of the ciliary body adjacent to the posterior Schwalbe ring. The underlying idea is to cause some tractional pull onto the trabecular region to open (at least, partly) the lumen of Schlemm's canal, which presumbly tends to collapse in open-angle glaucoma (NESTEROV et al.). The procedure of laser goniospasis is quite harmless and often results in some improvement in outflow facility. More time and experience are, however, necessary for a balanced assessment of the clinical value of this new procedure.

New fields for investigation can be opened up with the use of pulsed argon lasers, doubled-neodymium lasers, dye lasers, etc. Newer laser systems can be made much less cumbersome (one of such systems, presently in use, is fully incorporated into a conventional slit-lamp). Whatever its present state, the laser treatment in glaucoma opens up new scopes that are quite different from traditional treatment methods.

References

(1) Hager, H.: Laser-trabeculo puncture. In: International Glaucoma Symposium. Albi, 1974. Etienue, R.; Paterson, G.D. (eds.). Paris, pp. 419-434. Diffusion Générale de Libraire France 1975

(2) Krasnov, M.M.: Role of the laser in treatment of glaucoma. In: Current diagnosis and management of chorioretinal disease. L'Esperance, A. (ed.), pp. 411-421. St. Louis: Mosby 1977

(3) Perkins, E.S.; Brown, N.A.P.: Laser treatment of glaucoma. In: International Glaucoma Symposium. Albi, 1974. Etienue, R.; Paterson, G.D. (eds.), pp. 405-415. Diffusion Générale de Libraire France 1975

(4) Spitznas, M.: Discussion. In: Current diagnosis and management of chorioretinal disease. L'Esperance, A. (ed.), pp. 421-422. St. Louis: Mosby 1977

(5) Wheeler, C.B.: Laser iridectomy. Phys. Med. Biol. 22, 1115-1135 (1977).

Recent Advances in Glaucoma Microsurgery

J. Draeger

Augenklinik Zentralkrankenhaus, St. Jürgenstraße, D-2800 Bremen, Germany (FRG)

Microsurgery has added a new dimension to anterior segment surgery. Amazingly enough, glaucoma surgery so far has not benefited too much from the new methods and technologies. This partly may be due to the fact that in glaucoma surgery we do not deal with the transparent media as cornea or lens, but partly also to the change in attitude toward glaucoma treatment generally.

Apart from the discussion about indication, medical or surgical treatment, no doubt microsurgery can also contribute a great deal to glaucoma surgery. This is true for chamber angle procedures as well as for filtering operations.

First of all, a few words about the equipment needed: a modern microscope especially designed for ocular microsurgery with an appropriate illumination system that allows the quick change from coaxial to oblique illumination and can also be tilted, especially for use in goniotomy. Microscopic observation is also indispensable for the assistant (Fig.1). For some cases, a beam-splitting system is useful tu guarantee the same sight line and visual field for the assistant. When operating with higher magnification, the surgical field may exceed the visual field. Lateral mobility of the surgical table can then be helpful, and manual adjustment of the microscope can thus be avoided.

For surface preparation, a magnification of 6 - 10 × is usually satisfactory, although magnification of 40 × is required to locate Schlemm's canal. For operations in the iridocorneal angle ab interno, magnifications of about 15× are usually enough. These different requirements for certain operations and particular phases demand a wide range of magnification possibilities. If zoom optics are used, the factor should be about 5×. When a Galilei changer is used, graduated transitions between 6 and 40× are desirable.

When using relatively high magnifications, a stable vibrationless suspension is mandatory. In our experience, a ceiling mounting is to be preferred. A floor tripod is always exposed to the danger of inadvertent disturbance. Since the surgeon's hands are usually fully occupied, particularly during difficult phases of the operations, remote control by foot pedal is desirable for different functions.

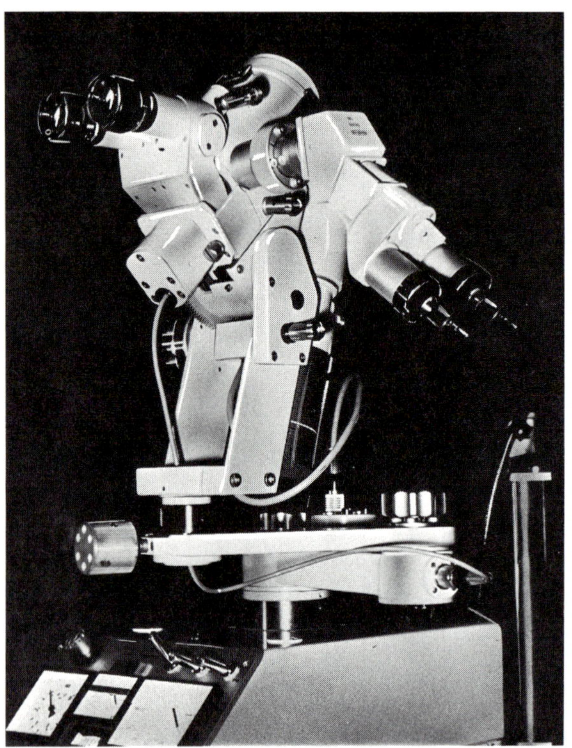

Fig.1. Assistant's microscope.

As far as specific operations are concerned, there have been some advances in instrumentation. Goniotomy only can be performed by use of concave contact lenses. Besides eliminating corneal reflection, they may add additional magnification due to their surface curvature. This type of lens designed by Barkan performs both the optical functions mentioned. If a suitable contact fluid is used, the total reflection is eliminated so that even if the eye piece is directed extremely tangentially, reflection free observation of the opposite angle is possible. The convex surface adds an additional magnification, which improves the depth of focus in the field.

New materials allow different design of the lens and make it more handsome (Fig. 2).

There are different models of microblades for goniotomy, with and without simultaneous irrigation. Experiments were also made with motorized microblades for goniotomy. The higher the cutting speed, the less cutting pressure is transmitted to the tissue. Increasing the cutting speed ten times means a decrease in cutting pressure by a tenth.

Following the same principle used for our rotary corneal trephine, another motorized rotating cutter was designed (Fig.3). A minute drill is protected in a small tube, which also provides the irrigation influx. The delicate incision can thus be performed without almost any pressure transmitted to the tissue surface.

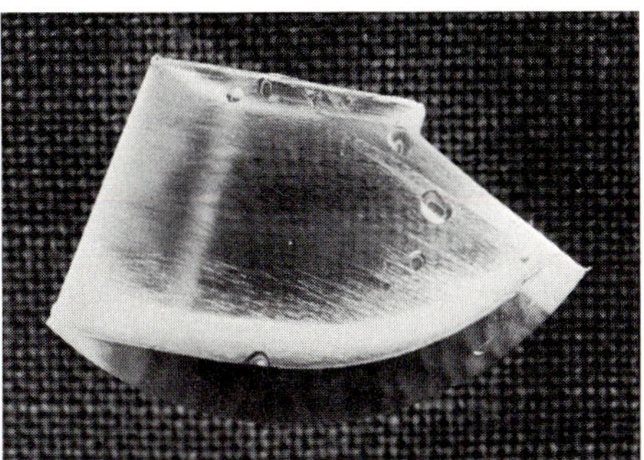

Fig.2. New silicone lens, lateral view.

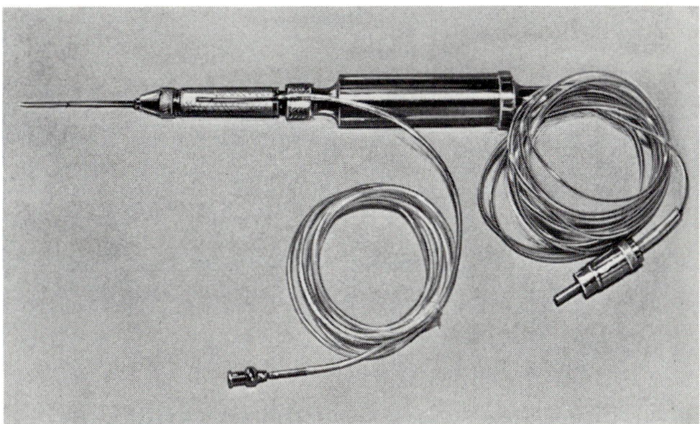

Fig.3. Motorized rotating microcutter.

For filtering procedures, Elliot's classic hand trephine was used, either for full thickness trepanation or for trepanation of the inner sceral layers. As in any other trepanation procedures, the cutting pressure on the tissue affects the curvature and consequently the edge of the cut. Convex or concave margins occur, frequently also more or less oblique canal sections, which as result of the unequal penetration of the cutting edge may endanger the structures lying behind it. For this reason, the rotary system mentioned can also be used with advantage for sceral trephination (Fig.4). The height of this instrument is very much less than that of the former manual instrument. Therefore, on vertical observation with coaxial illumination, one can even see the bottom of the trephine and the scleral surface. The moment of penetration can be assessed better than with manual trephination, in which the fingertips of the surgeon usually also complicate the view. For other phases of this operation, motorized cutting can also be used.

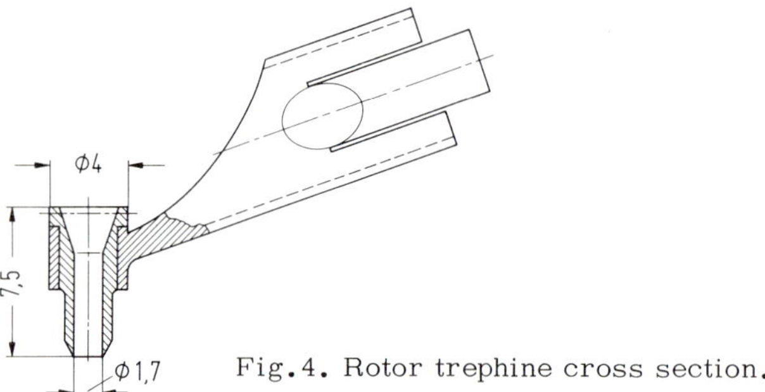

Fig.4. Rotor trephine cross section.

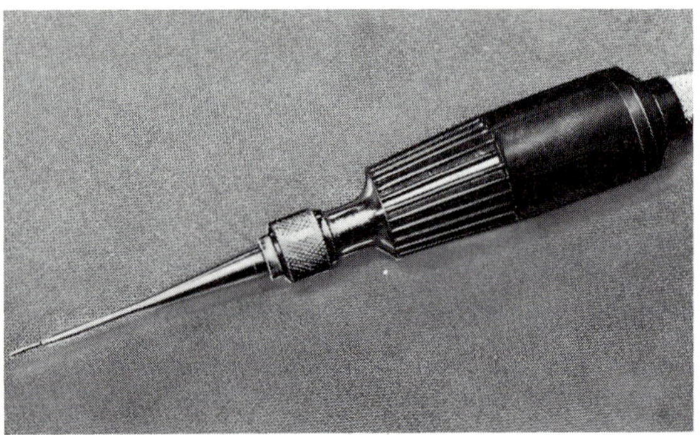

Fig.5. Rotor keratome, driven by air motor.

To preplace a limbal incision for later air injection we use a rotary keratome. To guarantee better reliability and higher torque, we have changed from electric motors to little air motors, providing five times the torque of an electric motor of the same size (Fig.5).

These few examples are to show that use of modern microsurgical technology also offers facilities for glaucoma microsurgery.

References

(1) Draeger, J.: Eine neue mikrochirurgische Operationseinheit. Vortragsband Jahrestagung 1968. Fortschr. Gebiet d. Neurochirurgie 92-96 (1969)

(2) Draeger, J.: Technique of goniotomy. Adv. Ophthalmol. 22, 183-184 (1970)

(3) Draeger, J.: Neue Schneidetechnik in der Mikrochirurgie. Klin. Mbl. Augenheilkd. 159, 293-303 (1972)

(4) Draeger, J.: Technische Fortschritte der Glaukombehandlung. Klin. Mbl. Augenheilkd. 163, 298-302 (1973)

(5) Draeger, J.: Optical equipment and instruments. In: Glaucomas. Heilmann, K.; Richardson, K.I. (eds.), pp. 313-317. Stuttgart: Thieme 1978

(6) Draeger, J.; Hackelbusch, R.: Experimentelle Untersuchungen und klinische Erfahrungen mit neuen Rotor-Instrumenten. Ophthalmologica 164, 273-283 (1972)

(7) Draeger, J.; Drecoll-Lütjen, E.; Rohen, W.: Histologische Untersuchungen über die strukturellen Veränderungen in der Kammerwinkelregion nach mikrochirurgischen Glaukom-Operationen. Klin. Mbl. Augenheilkd. 160, 281-291 (1972).

Discussion

KOLKER: I do not think that this discussion of glaucoma surgery should be completed without some mention of the concept of Schlemm's canal collapse (NESTEROV) as the possible etiology of the impaired outflow in open-angle glaucoma. In this regard, the goniospasis procedure of Cairns should be mentioned. If this concept is proved, it is possible that all of the procedures now used and described today may be discarded completely in the future.

LEE: 1) Utilizing Dr. J. RICE's technique, we have been successful in producing an effective pressure reduction in an eye with advanced open-angle glaucoma.
2) Transcorneal argon laser photocoagulation of the ciliary process is helpful and should be considered in carefully selected cases of aphakic glaucoma and malignant (aphakic) glaucoma or ciliary block glaucoma either as adjunct to medical or surgical management. The attractiveness of this procedure as a technique is of a surgical nature, but it is also non invasive, effective, and carries a low risk. Two cases were presented.

KRASNOV: I discussed the results of thermal (argon gas) goniopuncture with Drs. Kupfer and Gaasterland on many occasions (National Eye Institute of the United States). Their results show very clearly that thermal lasers should not be used (or used with special precautions) for goniopuncture because they cause serious inflammatory response with subsequent cicatrization closing the created channels of outflow. That is exactly why the work with short-pulsed, especially, Q-switched lasers, had been started.

Note added in proof: „Closing remarks" see page 212 „Epilogue"

Epilogue

W. Leydhecker

Immediately after the symposium and again after editing the discussion, I felt I should give my very personal impressions, instead of a balanced summary, as it was read to the International Congress of Ophthalmology. What were my lasting impressions? First, and most important of all, it was the atmosphere of friendship and co-operation that developed during these few days even with colleagues who had never met before. This requires good will and mutual esteem of all participants, but it can develop only in a small group of experts who number less than 40 individuals. In larger groups, there will be less freedom for discussions and more between speaker and auditory. In such small groups of experts only, the honesty to report on enormous work that unfortunately gave little positive results will be duly appreciated.
My second lasting impression regarded the vagaries of all present scientific glaucoma concepts. Fifteen years ago, it seemed clear that glaucoma was mainly a matter of the increased pressure, and the reason of pressure increase was a low facility of outflow. All these data could be measured. Some years later, the cup/disk ratio seemed to be the ground upon which to tread, with the consequence that a fundus camera might solve many of our clinical problems. And now - where are we? The difficulties and errors in measuring the intraocular pressure, the visual field, or the cup/disk ratio became evident. It was not even universally accepted how the cup/disk ratio is to be estimated or defined - does the cup start at the beginning of the slope or is it the area of pallor at the bottom of the slope? What does intraocular pressure mean at all, if 20 mm Hg can be associated with field defects, while 30 mm Hg does not matter in other eyes? Is glaucoma a matter of outflow pressure or a breakdown of auto regulation or an axoplasmic flow impediment? And what does any such statement signify clinically? It seemed uncertain that pressure regulation really stopped the field deterioration, but it seemed certain that miotics or surgery can produce or enhance cataract. This occurs especially in old patients, and there are insufficient intraindividual studies with only one eye treated or operated upon. Tension tolerance cannot be measured or even estimated with some degree of accuracy. It seemed impossible to separate eyes with ocular hypertension

from eyes with beginning glaucoma. Everything seemed vague, nowhere was there a firm ground to stand upon. This was one of the reasons why everyone was evasive in the final discussion.

Sure, there is no magic number for pressure that would separate normals from glaucoma or that calls for treatment. Agreed, there is no uniformly accepted way to describe the optic disk, and perhaps any number for the cup/disk ratio is less useful than a description or a drawing or a photograph. And fields - there are spontaneous variations, and everyone who ever did fields knows about the variability in the same patient, depending both on the observer and the patients present concentration and beginning cataract. Two more reasons for not committing oneself to any line of action seemed to be present: non commitment for the present time because in future we might have to admit errors and to change our ideas and non commitment because of fear of legal consequences.

I object to the non commitment for the time being. We have an obligation toward those who want a guideline in practice. It is a matter of course that we will have to change our ideas in the future. As regards fear of legal consequences, this is a very difficult situation in some countries, giving the patients the disadvantage of a doctor who has to think more about his own safety than about the benefit of the patient, a benefit that is often not available without some risk.

The third impression that struck me was that - strangely enough - in all discussions at Nara inside and outside the lecture hall it became clear that the participants manage glaucoma in a very similar manner. Evidently, the insecurities in theory cannot lift from our shoulders the clinical responsibility toward the individual patient who wants advice and a decision, right + here on the spot. I feel we should be less timid to state what our own guideline of action is at present, which can never be a canonic answer and should not include any obligation for others to do the same if they choose a different line of diagnosis or treatment.

I do not think we shall be able to find a magic number pertinent to each individual, but we should try to find the way back to numeric descriptions to define more precisely how and why we decide in practice. We must get away from vaguries without erroneously creating magic numbers. If a picture of a disk means something at all - as we all think it does - we should attempt to describe this picture in numbers. If we do tonometry at all - and certainly we all do - the result and its significance can be expressed in numbers. There is no science without numbers and measurements. Numbers are not magic, but they can be signs that make a bell ring in the doctor's head to do something in diagnosis or treatment.

What should he do? At present, it seems that the advice of experts is as vague as the diagnostic concept. They tell him to watch or to follow up if the intraocular pressure is below 30 mm Hg, perhaps even if it is higher, and in medical therapy or surgery the advice is not much more definite. This advice seems to me not very helpful in practice. We should specify what exactly should be done when, which brings us back to numbers or signs. I do not so much believe in divining in medicine but would trust more in defining conditions. We must not allow non medical people to play the controversies and insecurities of theoretic background against the reality of the consulting room. Comparatively speaking, we are like a musician who has to play an instrument even if he cannot explain in detail how it works. In our discussions at a symposium, we must have the freedom to ask the most heretic questions. But we cannot accept that such discussions are used against our clinical actions. We cannot allow non medical people to manipulate us into a diagnostic or therapeutic nihilism. This would be the end of healing.

Controversies in science and also an attempt to agree on practical lines might be one of the interesting subjects of the next meeting of the International Glaucoma Society in San Francisco in 1982.

Subject Index

Springer Books on Ophthalmology

Recent Advances in Glaucoma I

International Glaucoma Symposium,
Prague 1976
Editors: S. Rehák, M. M. Krasnov,
G. D. Paterson
1977. 77 figures, 46 tables.
XIII, 295 pages.
ISBN 3-540-07944-0
Distribution rights for the Socialist countries: Avicenum, Verlag für Medizin, Prague

S. N. Hassani

Real Time Ophthalmic Ultrasonography

1978. 423 figures. XXI, 214 pages.
ISBN 3-540-90318-6

Current Research in Ophthalmic Electron Microscopy

Editor: M. Spitznas
1977. 132 figures. VI, 183 pages.
ISBN 3-540-08508-4

S. S. Hayreh

Anterior Ischemic Optic Neuropathy

1975. 139 figures and 16 stereoscopic Illustrations. VIII, 145 pages.
ISBN 3-540-06916-X

G. Eisner

Biomicroscopy of the Peripheral Fundus

An Atlas and Textbook
Foreword by H. Goldmann.
Drawings by W. Hess.
1973. 121 figures, some in color.
XI, 191 pages.
ISBN 3-540-06374-9

Handbook of Sensory Physiology

Editorial Board: H. Autrum, R. Jung, W. R. Loewenstein, D. M. MacKay, H. L. Teuber

Volume 7
Part 3

Central Processing of Visual Information

Editor R. Jung

A: Integrative Functions and Comparative Data. 1973. 208 figures. XI, 775 pages.
ISBN 3-540-05769-2

B: Visual Centers in the Brain. 1973.
216 figures. VIII, 738 pages.
ISBN 3-540-06056-1

Part 1:

Photochemistry of Vision

Editor: H. J. A. Dartnall
1972. 296 figures. XII, 810 pages.
ISBN 3-540-05145-7

Part 2:

Physiology of Photoreceptor Organs

Editor: M. G. F. Fuortes
1972. 342 figures. X, 765 pages.
ISBN 3-540-05743-9

Visual Psychophysics

Editors: D. Jameson, L. M. Hurvich
1972. 297 figures. X, 812 pages.
ISBN 3-540-05146-5

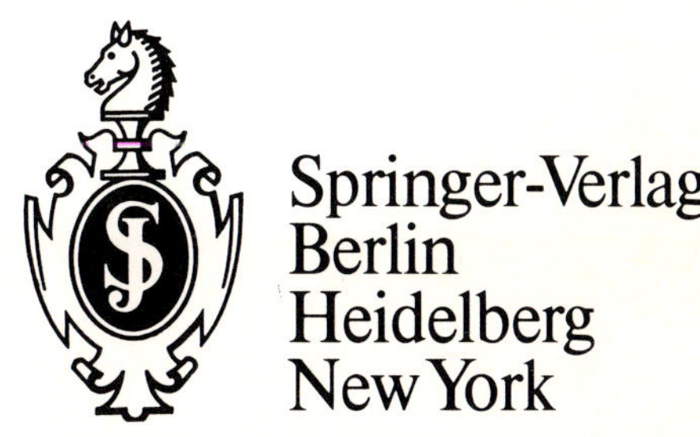

Neural Principles in Vision

Editors: G. Zettler, R. Weiler
1976. 293 figures. X, 430 pages.
(Proceedings in Life Sciences)
ISBN 3-540-07839-8

Augenbewegungsstörungen. Neurophysiologie und Klinik

(Disorders of Ocular Motility. Neurophysiological and Clinical Aspects).
Symposium der Deutschen Ophthalmologischen Gesellschaft vom 15.–17. April 1977 in Freiburg.
Herausgeber: G. Kommerell
1978. 182 Abbildungen, 49 Tabellen.
XVI, 382 Seiten (58 pages in English)
J. F. Bergmann Verlag, München
ISBN 3-8070-0303-7

Berichte über die Zusammenkünfte der Deutschen Ophthalmologischen Gesellschaft

74. Band

Periphere Retina

74. Zusammenkunft in Essen 1975.
Redigiert von W. Jaeger
1977. 714 Abbildungen, 78 Tabellen.
X, 934 Seiten
J. F. Bergmann Verlag, München
ISBN 3-8070-0297-9

75. Band

Kunststoffimplantate in der Opthalmologie

Redigiert von W. Jaeger
1978. 601 Abbildungen, 111 Tabellen.
XIII, 717 Seiten.
J. F. Bergmann Verlag, München
ISBN 3-8070-0304-5

G. Eisner

Augenchirurgie

Einführung in die operative Technik.
Einleitung: P. Niesel
Zeichnungen: P. Schneider
1978. 343 Abbildungen. XII, 184 Seiten.
ISBN 3-540-08371-5

Intraokularer Fremdkörper und Metallose

Internationales Symposium der Deutschen Ophthalmologischen Gesellschaft vom 30. März bis 2. April 1976 in Köln.
Herausgeber: H. Neubauer, W. Rüssmann, H. Kilp
1977. 229 Abbildungen, 70 Tabellen.
XVI, 470 Seiten (73 pages in English, 17 pages in French)
J. F. Bergmann Verlag, München
ISBN 3-8070-0301-0

W. Leydhecker

Manual der Tonographie für die Praxis

1977. 84 Abbildungen, 4 Tabellen, 2 Ausklapptafeln. VII, 115 Seiten.
(Kliniktaschenbücher)
ISBN 3-540-08093-7

W. Leydhecker, A. Kollmannsberger

Augenheilkunde. Neurologie

1978. 56 Abbildungen, 6 Tabellen.
XII, 180 Seiten. (Taschenbücher Allgemeinmedizin)
ISBN 3-540-08514-9

Therapie in der Augenheilkunde

Von E. Aulhorn, W. Böke, D. Friedburg, W. Leydhecker, O.-E. Lund, H. Neubauer, A. Nover, H. Pau, H.-J. Thiel, R. Witmer, J. Wollensak
Herausgeber: H. Pau
1977. 3 Abbildungen, 9 Tabellen.
XIX, 279 Seiten.
ISBN 3-540-08320-0

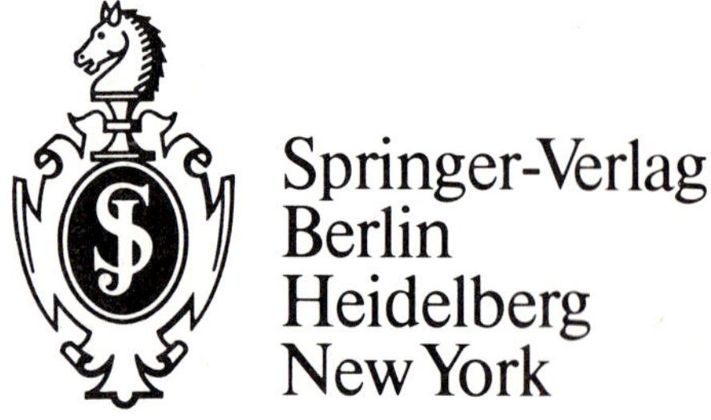